Pocket Guide to Pediatrics

Fifth Edition

Editor
William Porter, RN, CFRN, EMT-P

Contributing Editors
Dawn Phipps, RN, CCRN, CEN
Michele Moore, RN, RRT

JONES AND BARTLETT PUBLISHERS
Sudbury, Massachusetts
BOSTON   TORONTO   LONDON   SINGAPORE

World Headquarters
Jones and Bartlett Publishers
40 Tall Pine Drive
Sudbury, MA 01776
978-443-5000
info@jbpub.com
www.jbpub.com

Jones and Bartlett Publishers
Canada
6339 Ormindale Way
Mississauga, Ontario L5V 1J2
Canada

Jones and Bartlett Publishers
International
Barb House, Barb Mews
London W6 7PA
United Kingdom

Production Credits
Executive Editor: Kevin Sullivan
Acquisitions Editor: Emily Ekle
Associate Editor: Amy Sibley
Editorial Assistant: Patricia Donnelly
Production Director: Amy Rose
Production Editor: Carolyn F. Rogers
Marketing Manager: Katrina Gosek
Manufacturing Buyer: Amy Bacus
Composition: Graphic World
Text Design: Anne Spencer
Cover Design: Kristin E. Ohlin
Cover Image: © Photos.com
Printing and Binding: Imago
Cover Printing: Imago

6048

Printed in China
11 10 09 08 07   10 9 8 7 6 5 4 3 2 1

Contents

It is important to note that though there is a correlation between age and body weight, the clinician should use the patient's weight when calculating dosages. The dosages within this edition are the usual doses for the pediatric patient and might not be appropriate for adult patients.

An infant is between the ages of 28 days and 1 year. A child is between the ages of 1 and 12 years.

Medications

Medications

Medications

GENERIC NAME Brand Name®

A:	Action	partial list
I:	**Indication**	partial list
C:	Contraindication	partial list
SE:	Side Effects	partial list
N:	Notation	
D:	**Dose**	**Pediatric** dose
AD:	Administration	

Many methods of administration exist. Be certain to follow your institution's policy and procedure.

ACETAMINOPHEN Tylenol®

A: Analgesic, antipyretic
I: **Fever, Pain**
C: Use with caution in children with G6PD deficiency.
N: Increased risk of hepatotoxicity may occur with high doses of acetaminophen and barbiturates, phenytoin, carmustine, carbamazepine.
D: **Neonate:** 10–15 mg/kg/dose PO/PR q 6–8 hours. **Pediatrics:** 10–15 mg/kg/dose PO/PR q 4–6 hours.

Dosing by Age (PO/PR q 4–6 hours)	
Age	**Dose**
0–3 months	40 mg/dose
4–11 months	80 mg/dose
12–24 months	120 mg/dose
2–3 years	160 mg/dose
4–5 years	240 mg/dose
6–8 years	320 mg/dose
9–10 years	400 mg/dose
11–12 years	480 mg/dose

ADENOSINE Adenocard®

A: Slows AV conduction
I: **Paroxysmal Supraventricular Tachycardia**
C: Atrial fibrillation, atrial flutter, VT, sick sinus syndrome, second- or third-degree AV block.
SE: Facial flushing, SOB, chest pressure, N, lightheadedness.
N: Monitor/record cardiac rhythm.
D: Initial dose: **0.1 mg/kg RAPID IV** bolus given within 1–2 seconds. Repeat bolus: 0.2 mg/kg rapid IV if initial dose does not eliminate PSVT within 1–2 minutes.

ALBUTEROL Proventil®, Ventolin®

- **A:** Bronchodilator
- **I:** **Bronchospasm**
- **SE:** Palpitations, bronchospasm, tremors.
- **N:** Action may last up to 6 hours.
- **D:** 0.5% solution: **0.03 cc/kg in 3 cc NS** via nebulizer. Maximum dose = 1 cc.

AMINOPHYLLINE

- **A:** Bronchodilator
- **I:** **Bronchospasm**
- **C:** Active peptic ulcer, seizure disorder unless controlled by anticonvulsants.
- **SE:** N/V, headache, palpitations, tachycardia, ventricular dysrhythmias, hypotension, flushing, tachypnea, irritability, muscle twitching.
- **N:** Monitor VS and cardiac rhythm.
- **D:** **Loading dose** for patients not currently on theophylline products: **5–6 mg/kg IV** slowly over 20–30 minutes. **Maintenance infusion:** neonate, 0.2 mg/kg/h; 1 month–1 year old, 0.2–0.9 mg/kg/h; 1–9 years old, 1 mg/kg/h; 9–6 years old, 0.8 mg/kg/h.

500 mg in 500 ml = 1 mg/ml	
Dose	**Infusion Rate**
10 mg/h	10 ml/h
15 mg/h	15 ml/h
20 mg/h	20 ml/h
25 mg/h	25 ml/h
30 mg/h	30 ml/h
35 mg/h	35 ml/h
40 mg/h	40 ml/h
45 mg/h	45 ml/h
50 mg/h	50 ml/h
55 mg/h	55 ml/h
60 mg/h	60 ml/h

AMIODARONE

- A: Antiarrhythmic
- I: **Ventricular Fibrillation, Ventricular Tachycardia**
- C: Severe sinus node dysfunction, marked sinus bradycardia, second- and third-degree AV block.
- SE: Anorexia, N/V, dizziness, paresthesias, ataxia, tremor.
- N: Long elimination half-life (40–55 days).
- **D: Loading dose: 5 mg/kg IV over 30 minutes followed by a continuous infusion starting at 5 mcg/kg/min.**

AMRINONE Inocor®

- A: Positive inotrope, potent vasodilator
- I: **Congestive Heart Failure**
- SE: Dysrhythmias, hypotension, N/V, diarrhea, nephrogenic diabetes insipidus.
- N: Monitor VS, I&O, PAWP, CO, central venous pressure, cardiac rhythm, fluids, electrolytes, and renal function.
- D: Initial dose: **1–1.5 mg/kg IV** undiluted over 10 minutes; repeat q 30 minutes prn up to 3 boluses. Maintenance dose: neonate, 3–5 mcg/kg/min; older child, 10 mcg/kg/min.

ATROPINE

A: Enhances AV conduction
I: **Asystole, Bradycardia**
SE: Tachydysrhythmias.
N: Follow PALS guidelines. Will dilate pupils. Rapid IV bolus.
D: **0.02 mg/kg IV, IO or 0.04 mg/kg ET**
Minimum dose = 0.1 mg.
Maximum dose = 0.5 mg in child, 1 mg in adolescent. May repeat every 5 minutes to a maximum total dose of 1 mg in child, 2 mg in adolescent.

CHARCOAL, Activated

A: Binds with a wide variety of substances and inhibits their GI absorption.
I: **PO Drug Overdose, Poisoning**
C: Acetaminophen overdose where Mucomyst® is used.
N: Adding agents to enhance taste may increase PO compliance. Preparations often include sorbitol. If sorbitol is used, monitor child for prolonged diarrhea.
D: **1 g/kg PO, NG.**

CHLORAL HYDRATE

A: Sedation
I: **Sedation**
C: Severe cardiac disease, renal or hepatic failure.
SE: Drowsiness, N, nightmares.
N: Onset within 30–60 minutes.
D: **5–15 mg/kg PO, PR.**
Maximum single dose = 1 g.
Maximum daily dose = 2 g.

DANTROLENE Dantrium®

- A: Skeletal muscle relaxant
- I: **Spasticity Secondary to Chronic Disorders**
(e.g., multiple sclerosis, cerebral palsy)
- C: Active hepatic disease, upper motor neuron
disorders.
- SE: Hepatitis, muscle weakness, drowsiness,
diarrhea, constipation, dizziness.
- N: Avoid extravasation. Monitor liver function
tests.
- **D: 1 mg/kg IV;** repeat until symptoms abate, up
to maximum total dose of 10 mg/kg.

DEXAMETHASONE Decadron®

- A: Decreases inflammation, suppresses immune
response, stimulates bone marrow
- I/D: **Cerebral Edema:** 0.5–1.5 mg/kg IV, then
0.05–0.125 mg/kg IV q 6 hours.
Croup: 0.25–0.5 mg/kg IM, IV, or PO q 6 hours.
Meningitis: 0.15 mg/kg q 6 hours for 4 days.
- C: Patient with systemic fungal infection. Use
cautiously in patients with GI ulceration, renal
disease, diabetes mellitus, or seizures.
- SE: Euphoria, insomnia, peptic ulcer, hypokalemia,
hyperglycemia.
- N: Avoid abrupt withdrawal. Monitor growth in
patients on long-term therapy. May mask or
exacerbate infections.
- AD: IV use: Infuse boluses over 1 minute.

DEXTROSE

- A: Elevates serum glucose
- I: **Hypoglycemia**
- N: Extravasation may cause tissue necrosis.
- **D: 0.25–0.5 g/kg IV.**
- AD: Use 10% or 25% solution.

DIAZEPAM Valium®

- A: Elevates seizure threshold, relaxes skeletal muscle.
- I: **Seizure**
- C: Hypotension.
- SE: Respiratory depression, hypotension, confusion.
- N: Maintain airway and ventilation. Monitor BP. Incompatible with all drugs. May irritate vein.
- **D: 0.25 mg/kg IV,** may repeat every 5–15 minutes for 2 doses. Maximum single dose = 5 mg in child under 5 years, 10 mg in child over 5 years. Rectal dose: 0.5 mg/kg; do not exceed 10 mg.
- AD: Infuse slowly in 0.5-mg increments. Titrate to effect.

DIGOXIN

A: Positive inotrope

I: **Heart Failure, Atrial Fibrillation, Atrial Flutter, Paroxysmal Supraventricular Tachycardia**

C: Bradycardia, ventricular fibrillation.

SE: Ventricular dysrhythmias, AV block, visual disturbances, fatigue, N, agitation.

N: Toxicity may produce rhythm disturbances, bradycardia, and blurred or yellow vision and develops more frequently in patients with renal impairment. Monitor cardiac rhythm.

D: **Neonate:** Loading dose = 0.035 mg/kg PO daily, divided q 8 hours.
IV loading dose = 0.02–0.03 mg/kg.
Maintenance dose = 0.01 mg/kg daily, divided q 12 hours.
Child, 1 month–2 years: Loading dose = 0.035–0.06 mg/kg PO daily, divided q 8 hours.
IV loading dose = 0.03–0.05 mg/kg.
Maintenance dose = 0.01–0.02 mg/kg PO daily, divided q 12 hours.
Child over 2 years: Loading dose = 0.02–0.04 mg/kg PO daily, divided q 8 hours.
IV loading dose = 0.015–0.035 mg/kg.
Maintenance dose = 0.012 mg/kg PO daily, divided q 12 hours.

AD: IV use: Infuse over 5 minutes.

DIPHENHYDRAMINE Benadryl®

- A: Inhibits histamine release
- I: **Allergic or Dystonic Reaction**
- C: Asthma.
- SE: Drowsiness, N, dry mouth.
- **D: 1–2 mg/kg PO** or SLOW **IV.**
  Maximum daily dose = 300 mg.

DOBUTAMINE Dobutrex®

- A: Increases myocardial contractility and stroke volume
- I: **Depressed Myocardial Contractility**
- C: Idiopathic hypertrophic subaortic stenosis.
- SE: Palpitations, dyspnea, N, headache. Increase in HR, BP, and PVCs.
- N: Monitor HR, BP. The infusion rate should be adjusted as needed to stabilize the patient's BP and perfusion.
- **D: 2–20 mcg/kg/min IV.**
- AD: 6× body weight in kg is the mg dose to be added to IV solution to make 100 ml. Then 1 ml/h delivers 1 mcg/kg/min.

DOPAMINE Intropin®

A: Action is dose related:
2–5 mcg/kg/min provides inotropic support and increases renal perfusion.
5–15 mcg/kg/min increases cardiac output and peripheral resistance.

I: **Hemodynamic Imbalances in Shock Syndrome**

C: Tachydysrhythmias, VF pheochromocytoma.

SE: Ectopic beats, tachycardia, dyspnea, headache, hypotension, bradycardia, vasoconstriction, N/V.

N: Monitor peripheral pulses, BP, urinary output. Hypovolemia, if present, should be corrected prior to administration. Extravasation may cause tissue necrosis. Due to its peripheral vasoconstrictive effects, high infusion rates of dopamine may produce extremity ischemia in the child with shock.

D: Starting dose: **2–5 mcg/kg/min IV.**

AD: 6× body weight in kg is the mg dose to be added to IV solution to make 100 ml. Then 1 ml/h delivers 1 mcg/kg/min.

EPINEPHRINE

- A: Cardiac stimulation
- I: **Asystole, Bradycardia, Ventricular Fibrillation**
- SE: Tachycardia, palpitations, anxiety.
- N: Follow PALS guidelines. Monitor HR, BP, cardiac rhythm.
- D: **Neonate:** 0.1–0.3 ml/kg of **1:10,000** solution IV, IO.

  Infant or child: 0.1 ml/kg of **1:10,000** solution IV, IO once; increase to 0.1 ml/kg of **1:1,000** solution IV, IO and repeat q 3–5 minutes. ET dose is 0.1 ml/kg of 1:1,000 solution.

EPINEPHRINE, Infusion

- A: Cardiac stimulation
- I: **Hypotension, Bradycardia**
- SE: Tachycardia, palpitations, anxiety.
- N: Follow PALS guidelines. Monitor HR, BP, cardiac rhythm. Titrate to clinical effect.
- D: **0.1–1 mcg/kg/min IV.**
- AD: 0.6× body weight in kg is the mg dose added to NS or D5W to make 100 ml. Then 1 ml/h delivers 0.1 mcg/kg/min.

EPINEPHRINE 1:1,000

- A: Stimulates sympathetic nervous system
- I: **Bronchospasm, Allergic Reaction**
- C: Coronary insufficiency.
- SE: Tachycardia, palpitations, anxiety.
- N: Monitor HR, BP.
- D: **0.01 ml/kg SC.** May repeat q 20 minutes up to 4 hours.

EPINEPHRINE SUSPENSION Sus-Phrine®

A: Stimulates sympathetic nervous system
I: **Bronchospasm, Allergic Reaction**
C: Coronary insufficiency.
SE: Tachycardia, palpitations, anxiety.
N: Monitor HR, BP.
D: 0.005 ml/kg of 1:200 SC.
  Maximum single dose = 0.15 cc.

EPINEPHRINE, Racemic 2.25%

A: Stimulates sympathetic nervous system
I: **Croup, Postextubation Stridor**
SE: Tachycardia, palpitations, anxiety.
N: Rebound response common.
D: 0.05 ml/kg/dose in 3 cc NS via nebulizer over
  15 minutes, prn up to q 2 hours.
  Maximum dose = 0.5 cc.

FENTANYL Sublimaze®

- A: Narcotic analgesic
- I: **Pain Control**
- C: Asthma, myasthenia gravis, significant respiratory depression.
- SE: Sedation, clouded sensorium, euphoria, hypotension, bradycardia, constipation.
- N: Onset: 1–2 minutes; peaks within 10 minutes.
- D: **1–2 mcg/kg IM or SLOW IV.**
  Continuous infusion: 1 mcg/kg/h, titrate to effect. Usual range: 1–3 mcg/kg/h.

500 mcg in 100 ml NS = 5 mcg/ml

Weight kg	Dosage mcg/kg/h									
	0.5	1	1.5	2	2.5	3	3.5	4	4.5	5
5	0.5	1	1.5	2	2.5	3	3.5	4	4.5	5
10	1	2	3	4	5	6	7	8	9	10
15	1.5	3	4.5	6	7.5	9	10.5	12	13.5	15
20	2	4	6	8	10	12	14	16	18	20
25	2.5	5	7.5	10	12.5	15	17.5	20	22.5	25
30	3	6	9	12	15	18	21	24	27	30
35	3.5	7	10.5	14	17.5	21	24.5	28	31.5	35
40	4	8	12	16	20	24	28	32	36	40
45	4.5	9	13.5	18	22.5	27	31.5	36	40.5	45
50	5	10	15	20	25	30	35	40	45	50

Infusion rate ml/h

FLUMAZENIL Romazicon®

A: Benzodiazepine receptor antagonist

I: **Benzodiazepine Overdose**

C: Cyclic antidepressant overdose, patients given a benzodiazepine to control a life-threatening condition (e.g., control of intracranial pressure or status epilepticus).

SE: Dizziness, sweating, anxiety, headache, N/V, abnormal vision, injection site pain.

N: Maintain airway and ventilation. Monitor for resedation: Effects of Romazicon® may wear off before benzodiazepine clears the body. Infuse within a large vein. Anticipate rapid onset.

D: **0.01 mg/kg IV** over 30 seconds.

FUROSEMIDE Lasix®

A: Loop diuretic, vasodilation

I: **Edema**

C: Anuria, hypokalemia, hepatic coma.

SE: Volume depletion, hypotension, dizziness, hypokalemia, hypocalcemia, hypomagnesemia, and transient deafness if IV injection is given too rapidly.

N: Monitor HR, BP, fluids, and electrolytes.

D: **1 mg/kg IV** over 1–2 minutes.

GLUCAGON

- A: Increases serum glucose by stimulating hepatic glycogenolysis
- I: **Hypoglycemia**
- SE: N/V, SOB, urticaria.
- N: Onset within 5–20 minutes.
  Consider giving PO carbohydrates to restore liver glycogen and prevent secondary hypoglycemic episode. Consider IV dextrose if patient does not respond to glucagon.
- D: **0.1 mg/kg SC, IM.**
- AD: Reconstitute with diluent provided. Do not mix with medication or saline solutions.

HEPARIN

- A: Inhibits coagulation
- I: **Venous Thrombosis, Pulmonary Embolism, Peripheral Arterial Embolism**
- C: Active bleeding, severe thrombocytopenia.
- SE: Bleeding, thrombocytopenia.
- N: Obtain baseline coagulation studies.
  Antidote = protamine sulfate 1%.
- D: **50 units/kg IV** bolus, followed by an infusion of 10–25 units/kg/h.

INSULIN, Regular

- A: Lowers serum glucose
- I: **Diabetic Ketoacidosis**
- SE: Hypoglycemia, allergic reaction.
- N: Monitor BP, I&O, serum potassium and glucose, urine ketones and glucose.
  Incompatible with Dilantin®.
- D: **0.075 units/kg IV,** followed by an infusion of 0.1 units/kg/h.
  Neonates: Start with one-fourth to one-half of above infusion rate.
- AD: 100 units in 100 ml IV solution = 1 U/ml.

KETAMINE Ketalar®

- A: Blocks pain perception
- I: **Sedation for Short-Term Procedures**
- C: Elevated ICP or intraocular pressure, hypertension, CHF, psychotic disorders.
- SE: Hypertension, hypotension, tachycardia, increased ICP and intraocular pressure, emergence reactions, laryngospasm, apnea, salivation, N/V.
- N: Onset IV: 30–120 seconds. Duration IV: 20–60 minutes. May premedicate with atropine to decrease salivation. Rate of IV infusion should not exceed 0.5 mg/kg/min.
- D: **IV: 0.25–0.5 mg/kg SLOWLY.**
  IM: 1.5–2 mg/kg.

LIDOCAINE

- A: Elevates ventricular fibrillation threshold
- I: **Ventricular Fibrillation, Ventricular Tachycardia**
- C: AV block, hypotension, bradycardia.
- SE: Toxicity: Drowsiness, disorientation, seizure, lightheadedness, decreased hearing ability, hypotension, paresthesias, muscle twitching.
- N: Monitor BP and cardiac rhythm.
- D: **1 mg/kg IV, IO or 2 mg/kg ET;** may repeat q 5–10 minutes.
  Maximum total dose = 3 mg/kg.
  IV infusion to follow bolus: 20–50 mcg/kg/min.

LORAZEPAM

- A: Sedation
- I: **Seizure**
- SE: Drowsiness, transient hypotension.
- N: Maintain airway and ventilation. Monitor BP.
- D: **0.05–0.1 mg/kg SLOW IV, deep IM or PR.**
- AD: IV use: Dilute 1:1 with D5W, NS, or SW.

MANNITOL, 20%

- A: Reduces ICP and cerebral edema
- I: **Severe Head Injury**
- C: Active intracranial bleeding, pulmonary edema, severe dehydration, anuria secondary to renal failure.
- SE: Edema, thrombophlebitis, hypotension, hypertension, N/V, headache, blurred vision, seizures, pulmonary congestion, acidosis, fluid and electrolyte imbalance, marked diuresis.
- N: Monitor VS, I&O. Do not mix with blood transfusions. Use in-line filter.
- D: **0.25–1 g/kg IV** over 10–15 minutes.

METHYLPREDNISOLONE Solu-Medrol®

A: Decreases inflammation

I/D: **Asthma:** 1–2 mg/kg IV once, followed by
0.5 mg/kg IV q 6 hours.
Acute Spinal Cord Injury: 30 mg/kg IV over
15 minutes, wait 45 minutes, then infuse
5.4 mg/kg/h × 23 hours.

C: Patients with systemic fungal infections. Use
cautiously in patients with GI ulceration, renal
disease, diabetes mellitus, or seizures.

SE: CHF, euphoria, insomnia, peptic ulcer,
hypokalemia, hyperglycemia, carbohydrate
intolerance, growth suppression.

N: Avoid abrupt withdrawal.

MIDAZOLAM Versed®

A: Depresses CNS

I: **Sedation**

C: Severe hypotension. Use cautiously in patients
with severe hepatic dysfunction, renal failure,
or CHF.

SE: Apnea, decreased respiratory rate.

N: Monitor for respiratory depression. Avoid
extravasation.

D: **0.075–0.15 mg/kg IM** or **SLOW IV.** Decrease
dose by 25% when narcotics are given
concurrently.
Maximum total dose = 0.2 mg/kg.

MORPHINE SULFATE

A: Potent narcotic analgesic
I: **Severe Pain**
SE: Respiratory depression, hypotension, sedation,
    clouded sensorium, euphoria, bradycardia,
    seizures, nightmares, N/V.
N: Monitor for respiratory depression.
D: **0.1–0.2 mg/kg IM** or **IV** over 5 minutes.

NALOXONE Narcan®

A: Narcotic antagonist
I: **Acute Narcotic Overdose**
N: Anticipate rapid onset.
    Neonates: Use 0.02 mg/ml concentration.
D: **Neonate–5 years:** 0.1 mg/kg IV, IM, ET, IO.
    Children 5 years and older: 2 mg IV, IM, ET, IO.

NIFEDIPINE Procardia®

A: Calcium channel blocker
I: **Hypertensive Crisis**
SE: Hypotension, dyspnea, peripheral edema,
    flushing, tachycardia, palpitations, headache.
D: **0.25–0.5 mg/kg PO, SL** q 6–8 hours.
AD: To withdraw capsule contents, puncture one
    end of capsule. Puncture opposite end and
    draw contents with needle and syringe.

NITROPRUSSIDE Nitropress®

A: Dilates peripheral arteries and veins

I: **Hypertensive Crisis**

C: Compensatory hypertension (i.e., arteriovenous shunt or coarctation of the aorta).

SE: N/V, diaphoresis, apprehension, headache, retrosternal discomfort, palpitations, muscle twitching.

N: Monitor and titrate to BP. Side effects are usually associated with rapid reduction in BP. Wrap container in aluminum foil to protect from light. Monitor serum thiocyanate levels in cases of prolonged use (> 48 hours). Do not mix with medications.

D: **0.1–10 mcg/kg/min IV.**

AD: $6\times$ body weight in kg is the mg dose to be added to IV solution to make 100 ml. Then 1 ml/h delivers 1 mcg/kg/min.

PANCURONIUM Pavulon®

A: Skeletal muscle relaxation and paralysis

I: **Facilitate Endotracheal Intubation**

SE: Apnea, tachycardia, salivation, transient rash, prolonged skeletal muscle relaxation.

N: **MUST BE ABLE TO VENTILATE PATIENT.**
Onset: 30–45 seconds. Peak: 3–5 minutes. Duration: 60 minutes.

D: **0.04–0.15 mg/kg IV.**
Defasciculating dose: 0.01 mg/kg IV.

PHENOBARBITAL

A: Depresses CNS; increases seizure threshold

I/D: **Status Epilepticus:** 10–20 mg/kg SLOW IV once, then 5–10 mg/kg q 20 minutes prn. Maximum total dose = 40 mg/kg.
Sedation: 6 mg/kg/24 hour PO, divided tid.

C: Hepatic or renal disease, porphyria.

SE: Stevens-Johnson syndrome, N/V, drowsiness, angioedema.

N: Monitor for respiratory depression and hypotension. Obtain VS prior to administration. Discard if solution contains a precipitate.

PHENYLEPHRINE Neo-Synephrine®

A: Stimulates sympathetic nervous system

I: **Severe Hypotension**

C: Tachydysrhythmias, fluid volume deficits.

SE: Hypertension, bradycardia, tachycardia, chest pain, headache, insomnia.

N: Monitor BP, cardiac rhythm. Correct volume depletion, if present, prior to administration. Extravasation at IV site should be treated promptly with 10–15 ml NS containing 5–10 mg phentolamine.

D: **5–20 mcg/kg/dose IV** q 10–15 minutes prn.
Continuous infusion: 0.1–0.5 mcg/kg/min; titrate to effect.

PHENYTOIN Dilantin®

A: Stabilizes neuronal membranes

I: **Seizures**

C: Sinus bradycardia, AV block, Adams-Stokes syndrome, seizure due to hypoglycemia. Use cautiously in presence of impaired renal or hepatic function, alcoholism, hypotension.

SE: Nystagmus, drowsiness, ataxia, bradycardia, VF, hypotension, photophobia, V, rash.

N: Mix with NS only. Use in-line filter. Avoid IM administration.

D: **10–20 mg/kg** SLOW **IV** infusion over 30 minutes, up to maximum dose of 1 g.

PROSTAGLANDIN E₁ Prostin VR®

A: Inhibits platelet aggregation

I: **Temporarily Maintain Patency of Ductus Arteriosus in Neonates.**
   Congenital Defects: Pulmonary Atresia, Pulmonary Stenosis, Tricuspid Atresia, Tetralogy of Fallot, Coarctation of the Aorta or Transposition of the Great Vessels.

SE: Apnea, fever, seizures, flushing, bradycardia, hypotension, diarrhea.

N: Monitor vital signs and arterial oxygen saturation closely. Infuse within a large vein.

D: Start at **0.05–0.1 mcg/kg/min IV.** Titrate. Use minimal dose necessary to maintain clinical response.

ROCURONIUM Zemuron®

A: Neuromuscular blocking agent
I: **Facilitate Endotracheal Intubation**
SE: Arrhythmia, tachycardia, N/V, rash, bronchospasm.
N: **MUST BE ABLE TO VENTILATE PATIENT.**
   Minimal cardiovascular effects. Peak effects occur in 0.5–1 minute. Duration: 30–40 minutes.
D: **0.6–1.2 mg/kg/dose × 1**, if needed; maintenance doses of 0.1–0.2 mg/kg/dose q 20–30 minutes.
AD: Continuous infusion: Start at 10–12 mcg/kg/min; titrate to effect.

SUCCINYLCHOLINE Anectine®

A: Skeletal muscle relaxation and paralysis
I: **Facilitate Endotracheal Intubation**
C: Acute narrow-angle glaucoma, penetrating eye injury, history of malignant hyperthermia.
SE: Bradycardia, tachycardia, cardiac arrest, hypotension, hypertension, malignant hyperthermia.
N: **MUST BE ABLE TO VENTILATE PATIENT.**
   Premedicate with atropine prior to intubation. Onset: 30–60 seconds. Duration: 2–3 minutes.
D: **1–2 mg/kg IV** over 10–30 seconds. May repeat 0.3–0.6 mg/kg in 5–10 minutes. Use larger doses in infants.
   IM use: 2–4 mg/kg prn.
   Maximum dose = 150 mg.

THIOPENTAL SODIUM Pentothal®

- A: Inhibits firing rate of neurons within ascending reticular-activating system.
- I: **Induce Anesthesia**
- C: Acute intermittent porphyria.
- SE: Prolonged somnolence, myocardial and respiratory depression, arrhythmias, bronchospasm, laryngospasm.
- N: Monitor for respiratory depression. Peak brain concentrations reached in 10–20 seconds; consciousness returns in 20–30 minutes.
- D: **4–5 mg/kg IV.**

VASOPRESSIN Pitressin®

- A: Promotes reabsorption of water
- I: **Non-nephrogenic Diabetes Insipidus**
- C: Chronic nephritis accompanied by nitrogen retention.
- SE: Anaphylaxis, hypertension, bradycardia, tremor, sweating, vertigo, N/V, urticaria.
- N: Monitor I&O. Observe for edema.
- D: **0.5 mU/kg/h IV.** Titrate to clinical response up to 15 mU/kg/h.

VECURONIUM Norcuron®

A: Skeletal muscle relaxation and paralysis

I: **Facilitate Endotracheal Intubation**

C: Aminoglycoside antibiotics, including amikacin, gentamicin, kanamycin, neomycin, streptomycin. Polymyxin antibiotics; clindamycin; quinidine. Halothane, enflurane, and isoflurane interact and potentiate neuromuscular blockade, leading to prolonged skeletal muscle relaxation.

SE: Apnea, prolonged skeletal muscle relaxation.

N: **MUST BE ABLE TO VENTILATE PATIENT.**
Minimal effect on cardiovascular system. No cumulative effects. Recovery prolonged by acidosis.
Onset: 1 minute. Peak: 3–5 minutes. Duration: 25–65 minutes.

D: **0.1–0.3 mg/kg IV.**

Instant Pediatric Doses

▮ Instant Pediatric Doses

It is important to note that though there is a correlation between age and body weight, the clinician should use the patient's true body weight when calculating dosages.

The following pages give you the **usual** body weight for a given age and calculate the appropriate dose and volumes for the medications described. Normal vital signs and sizes of equipment/supplies are also listed.

Wt (kg) Age		Heart rate (beats per minute) Respiratory rate (breaths per minute) Systolic blood pressure (mmHg)	
Drug	**Dose**	**Deliver mg**	**Deliver cc**

Fluid challenge: 20 ml/kg NS or LR, IV or IO*

Equipment

ETT (mm)   Foley (Fr)
ETT @ lip (cm)   Chest tube (Fr)
NG tube (Fr)   Suction cath (Fr)

* Neonates receive 10 ml/kg.

3 kg Term		Heart rate	125
		Respiratory rate	60
		Systolic BP	70

Drug	Dose	Deliver (mg)	Deliver (cc)
Atropine 0.1 mg/cc	0.02 mg/kg IV, IO, ET	0.06 mg	► 0.6 cc
Dextrose 10% 0.10 g/cc	0.5 g/kg IV, IO	1.5 g	► 15 cc
Epinephrine 1:10,000	0.01 mg/kg IV, IO	0.03 mg	► 0.3 cc
Ketamine	1–2 mg/kg IV, IO	3–6 mg	
Lorazepam 2 mg/cc	0.05–0.1 mg/kg IV, IO, IM	0.5–0.3 mg	► 0.075–0.15 cc
Midazolam 1 mg/cc	0.05–0.1 mg/kg IV, IO	0.15–0.3 mg	► 0.15–0.3 cc
Rocuronium 10 mg/cc	0.6 mg/kg IV bolus	1.8 mg	► 0.18 cc

Fluid challenge: 30 ml NS or LR

Equipment

ETT	3 mm	Foley	6 Fr
ETT @ lip	9 cm	Chest tube	12 Fr
NG tube	5–8 Fr	Suction cath	8 Fr

Defibrillation: 6 J, 12 J, 12 J (2 J/kg, 4 J/kg, 4 J/kg)
Cardioversion: 1.5 J (0.5 J/kg)

6 kg 3 mo		Heart rate	125
		Respiratory rate	36–48
		Systolic BP	80 ± 20

Drug	Dose	Deliver (mg)	Deliver (cc)
Atropine 0.1 mg/cc	0.02 mg/kg IV, IO, ET	0.12 mg	▶ 1.2 cc
Dextrose 25% 0.25 g/cc	0.5 g/kg IV, IO	3 g	▶ 12 cc
Epinephrine 1:10,000	0.01 mg/kg IV, IO	0.06 mg	▶ 0.6 cc
Ketamine	1–2 mg/kg IV, IO	6–12 mg	
Lorazepam 2 mg/cc	0.05–0.1 mg/kg IV, IO	0.3–0.6 mg	▶ 0.15–0.3 cc
Midazolam 1 mg/cc	0.05–0.1 mg/kg IV, IO	0.3–0.6 mg	▶ 0.3–0.6 cc
Rocuronium 10 mg/cc	0.6 mg/kg IV bolus	3.6 mg	▶ 0.36 cc

Fluid challenge: 120 ml NS or LR

Equipment

ETT	3–3.5 mm	Foley	6 Fr
ETT @ lip	11 cm	Chest tube	12 Fr
NG tube	8 Fr	Suction cath	8 Fr

Defibrillation: 12 J, 24 J, 24 J (2 J/kg, 4 J/kg, 4 J/kg)
Cardioversion: 3 J (0.5 J/kg)

7 kg	Heart rate	120
6 mo	Respiratory rate	24–36
	Systolic BP	90 ± 30

Drug	Dose	Deliver (mg)	Deliver (cc)
Atropine 0.1 mg/cc	0.02 mg/kg IV, IO, ET	0.14 mg	▶ 1.4 cc
Dextrose 25% 0.25 g/cc	0.5 g/kg IV, IO	3.5 g	▶ 14 cc
Epinephrine 1:10,000	0.01 mg/kg IV, IO	0.07 mg	▶ 0.7 cc
Ketamine	1–2 mg/kg IV, IO	7–14 mg	
Lorazepam 2 mg/cc	0.05–0.1 mg/kg IV, IO	0.35–0.7 mg	▶ 0.175–0.35 cc
Midazolam 1 mg/cc	0.05–0.1 mg/kg IV, IO	0.35–0.7 mg	▶ 0.35–0.7 cc
Rocuronium 10 mg/cc	0.6 mg/kg IV bolus	4.2 mg	▶ 0.42 cc

Fluid challenge: 140 ml NS or LR

Equipment

ETT	3.5–4 mm	Foley	6 Fr
ETT @ lip	11 cm	Chest tube	12–16 Fr
NG tube	8 Fr	Suction cath	8 Fr

Defibrillation: 14 J, 28 J, 28 J (2 J/kg, 4 J/kg, 4 J/kg)
Cardioversion: 3.5 J (0.5 J/kg)

8.5 kg		Heart rate	120
9 mo		Respiratory rate	24–32
		Systolic BP	92 ± 30

Drug	Dose	Deliver (mg)	Deliver (cc)
Atropine 0.1 mg/cc	0.02 mg/kg IV, IO, ET	0.17 mg	▶ 1.7 cc
Dextrose 25% 0.25 g/cc	0.5 g/kg IV, IO	4.25 g	▶ 17 cc
Epinephrine 1:10,000	0.01 mg/kg IV, IO	0.085 mg	▶ 0.85 cc
Ketamine	1–2 mg/kg IV, IO	8.5–17 mg	
Lorazepam 2 mg/cc	0.05–0.1 mg/kg IV, IO	0.42–0.85 mg	▶ 0.21–0.42 cc
Midazolam 1 mg/cc	0.05–0.1 mg/kg IV, IO	0.42–0.85 mg	▶ 0.42–0.85 cc
Rocuronium 10 mg/cc	0.6 mg/kg IV bolus	5.1 mg	▶ 0.51 cc

Fluid challenge: 170 ml NS or LR

Equipment

ETT	3.5–4 mm	Foley	6–8 Fr
ETT @ lip	11 cm	Chest tube	16 Fr
NG tube	8 Fr	Suction cath	8 Fr

Defibrillation: 17 J, 34 J, 34 J (2 J/kg, 4 J/kg, 4 J/kg)
Cardioversion: 4.25 J (0.5 J/kg)

10 kg 1 y		Heart rate	120
		Respiratory rate	24–32
		Systolic BP	92 ± 30

Drug	Dose	Deliver (mg)	Deliver (cc)
Atropine 0.1 mg/cc	0.02 mg/kg IV, IO, ET	0.2 mg	▶ 2 cc
Dextrose 25% 0.25 g/cc	0.5 g/kg IV, IO	5 g	▶ 20 cc
Epinephrine 1:10,000	0.01 mg/kg IV, IO	0.1 mg	▶ 1 cc
Ketamine	1–2 mg/kg IV, IO	10–20 mg	
Lorazepam 2 mg/cc	0.05–0.1 mg/kg IV, IO	0.5–1 mg	▶ 0.25–0.5 cc
Midazolam 1 mg/cc	0.05–0.1 mg/kg IV, IO	0.5–1 mg	▶ 0.5–1 cc
Rocuronium 10 mg/cc	0.6 mg/kg IV bolus	6 mg	▶ 0.6 cc

Fluid challenge: 200 ml NS or LR

Equipment

ETT	4–4.5 mm	Foley	8 Fr
ETT @ lip	11 cm	Chest tube	20 Fr
NG tube	8 Fr	Suction cath	8 Fr

Defibrillation: 20 J, 40 J, 40 J (2 J/kg, 4 J/kg, 4 J/kg)
Cardioversion: 5 J (0.5 J/kg)

11 kg		Heart rate	115
18 mo		Respiratory rate	22–28
		Systolic BP	96 ± 30

Drug	Dose	Deliver (mg)	Deliver (cc)
Atropine 0.1 mg/cc	0.02 mg/kg IV, IO, ET	0.22 mg	▶ 2.2 cc
Dextrose 25% 0.25 g/cc	0.5 g/kg IV, IO	5.5 g	▶ 22 cc
Epinephrine 1:10,000	0.01 mg/kg IV, IO	0.11 mg	▶ 1.1 cc
Ketamine	1–2 mg/kg IV, IO	11–22 mg	
Lorazepam 2 mg/cc	0.05–0.1 mg/kg IV, IO	0.5–1.1 mg	▶ 0.25–0.55 cc
Midazolam 1 mg/cc	0.05–0.1 mg/kg IV, IO	0.5–1.1 mg	▶ 0.5–1.1 cc
Rocuronium 10 mg/cc	0.6 mg/kg IV bolus	6.6 mg	▶ 0.66 cc

Fluid challenge: 220 ml NS or LR

Equipment

ETT	4–4.5 mm	Foley	8 Fr
ETT @ lip	12 cm	Chest tube	20 Fr
NG tube	8 Fr	Suction cath	8 Fr

Defibrillation: 22 J, 44 J, 44 J (2 J/kg, 4 J/kg, 4 J/kg)
Cardioversion: 5.5 J (0.5 J/kg)

12 kg		Heart rate	115
2 y		Respiratory rate	22–28
		Systolic BP	98 ± 30

Drug	Dose	Deliver (mg)	Deliver (cc)
Atropine 0.1 mg/cc	0.02 mg/kg IV, IO, ET	0.24 mg	► 2.4 cc
Dextrose 50% 0.5 g/cc	0.5 g/kg IV, IO	6 g	► 12 cc
Epinephrine 1:10,000	0.01 mg/kg IV, IO	0.12 mg	► 1.2 cc
Ketamine	1–2 mg/kg IV, IO	12–24 mg	
Lorazepam 2 mg/cc	0.05–0.1 mg/kg IV, IO	0.6–1.2 mg	► 0.3–0.6 cc
Midazolam 1 mg/cc	0.05–0.1 mg/kg IV, IO	0.6–1.2 mg	► 0.6–1.2 cc
Rocuronium 10 mg/cc	0.6 mg/kg IV bolus	7.2 mg	► 0.72 cc

Fluid challenge: 240 ml NS or LR

Equipment

ETT	4–4.5 mm	Foley	8 Fr
ETT @ lip	12 cm	Chest tube	20–24 Fr
NG tube	10 Fr	Suction cath	8 Fr

Defibrillation: 24 J, 48 J, 48 J (2 J/kg, 4 J/kg, 4 J/kg)
Cardioversion: 6 J (0.5 J/kg)

14 kg		Heart rate	110
3 y		Respiratory rate	20–26
		Systolic BP	100 ± 25

Drug	Dose	Deliver (mg)	Deliver (cc)
Atropine 0.1 mg/cc	0.02 mg/kg IV, IO, ET	0.28 mg	▶ 2.8 cc
Dextrose 50% 0.5 g/cc	0.5 g/kg IV, IO	7 g	▶ 14 cc
Epinephrine 1:10,000	0.01 mg/kg IV, IO	0.14 mg	▶ 1.4 cc
Ketamine	1–2 mg/kg IV, IO	14–28 mg	
Lorazepam 2 mg/cc	0.05–0.1 mg/kg IV, IO	0.7–1.4 mg	▶ 0.35–0.7 cc
Midazolam 1 mg/cc	0.05–0.1 mg/kg IV, IO	0.7–1.4 mg	▶ 0.7–1.4 cc
Rocuronium 10 mg/cc	0.6 mg/kg IV bolus	8.4 mg	▶ 0.84 cc

Fluid challenge: 280 ml NS or LR

Equipment

ETT	4.5–5 mm	Foley	8–10 Fr
ETT @ lip	13 cm	Chest tube	20–24 Fr
NG tube	10 Fr	Suction cath	10 Fr

Defibrillation: 28 J, 56 J, 56 J (2 J/kg, 4 J/kg, 4 J/kg)
Cardioversion: 7 J (0.5 J/kg)

16 kg		Heart rate	105
4 y		Respiratory rate	20–26
		Systolic BP	100 ± 22

Drug	Dose	Deliver (mg)	Deliver (cc)
Atropine	0.02 mg/kg	0.32 mg	▶ 3.2 cc
0.1 mg/cc	IV, IO, ET		
Dextrose 50%	0.5 g/kg	8 g	▶ 16 cc
0.5 g/cc	IV, IO		
Epinephrine	0.01 mg/kg	0.16 mg	▶ 1.6 cc
1:10,000	IV, IO		
Ketamine	1–2 mg/kg	16–32 mg	
	IV, IO		
Lorazepam	0.05–0.1 mg/kg	0.8–1.6 mg	▶ 0.4–0.8 cc
2 mg/cc	IV, IO		
Midazolam	0.05–0.1 mg/kg	0.8–1.6 mg	▶ 0.8–1.6 cc
1 mg/cc	IV, IO		
Rocuronium	0.6 mg/kg	10 mg	▶ 1 cc
10 mg/cc	IV bolus		

Fluid challenge: 320 ml NS or LR

Equipment

ETT	4.5–5 mm	Foley	10 Fr
ETT @ lip	13 cm	Chest tube	24 Fr
NG tube	10 Fr	Suction cath	10 Fr

Defibrillation: 32 J, 64 J, 64 J (2 J/kg, 4 J/kg, 4 J/kg)
Cardioversion: 8 J (0.5 J/kg)

18 kg		Heart rate	100
5 y		Respiratory rate	20–24
		Systolic BP	100 ± 22

Drug	Dose	Deliver (mg)	Deliver (cc)
Atropine 0.1 mg/cc	0.02 mg/kg IV, IO, ET	0.36 mg	► 3.6 cc
Dextrose 50% 0.5 g/cc	0.5 g/kg IV, IO	9 g	► 18 cc
Epinephrine 1:10,000	0.01 mg/kg IV, IO	0.18 mg	► 1.8 cc
Ketamine	1–2 mg/kg IV, IO	18–36 mg	
Lorazepam 2 mg/cc	0.05–0.1 mg/kg IV, IO	0.9–1.8 mg	► 0.45–0.9 cc
Midazolam 1 mg/cc	0.05–0.1 mg/kg IV, IO	0.9–1.8 mg	► 0.9–1.8 cc
Rocuronium 10 mg/cc	0.6 mg/kg IV bolus	11 mg	► 1.1 cc

Fluid challenge: 360 ml NS or LR

Equipment

ETT	5–5.5 mm	Foley	10 Fr
ETT @ lip	14 cm	Chest tube	24 Fr
NG tube	10 Fr	Suction cath	10 Fr

Defibrillation: 36 J, 72 J, 72 J (2 J/kg, 4 J/kg, 4 J/kg)
Cardioversion: 9 J (0.5 J/kg)

20 kg		Heart rate	100
6 y		Respiratory rate	20–24
		Systolic BP	100 ± 15

Drug	Dose	Deliver mg	Deliver cc
Atropine	0.02 mg/kg	0.4 mg	▶ 4 cc
0.1 mg/cc	IV, IO, ET		
Dextrose 50%	0.5 g/kg	10 g	▶ 20 cc
0.5 g/cc	IV, IO		
Epinephrine	0.01 mg/kg	0.2 mg	▶ 2 cc
1:10,000	IV, IO		
Ketamine	1–2 mg/kg	20–40 mg	
	IV, IO		
Lorazepam	0.05–0.1 mg/kg	1–2 mg	▶ 0.5–1 cc
2 mg/cc	IV, IO		
Midazolam	0.05–0.1 mg/kg	1–2 mg	▶ 1–2 cc
1 mg/cc	IV, IO		
Rocuronium	0.6 mg/kg	12 mg	▶ 1.2 cc
10 mg/cc	IV bolus		

Fluid challenge: 400 ml NS or LR

Equipment

ETT	5–5.5 mm	Foley	10 Fr
ETT @ lip	15 cm	Chest tube	28 Fr
NG tube	12 Fr	Suction cath	10 Fr

Defibrillation: 40 J, 80 J, 80 J (2 J/kg, 4 J/kg, 4 J/kg)
Cardioversion: 10 J (0.5 J/kg)

24 kg		Heart rate	90	
8 y		Respiratory rate	18–22	
		Systolic BP	105 ± 15	

Drug	Dose	Deliver (mg)	Deliver (cc)
Atropine 0.1 mg/cc	0.02 mg/kg IV, IO, ET	0.48 mg	▶ 4.8 cc
Dextrose 50% 0.5 g/cc	0.5 g/kg IV, IO	12 g	▶ 24 cc
Epinephrine 1:10,000	0.01 mg/kg IV, IO	0.24 mg	▶ 2.4 cc
Ketamine	1–2 mg/kg IV, IO	24–48 mg	
Lorazepam 2 mg/cc	0.05–0.1 mg/kg IV, IO	1.2–2.4 mg	▶ 0.6–1.2 cc
Midazolam 1 mg/cc	0.05–0.1 mg/kg IV, IO	1.2–2.4 mg	▶ 1.2–2.4 cc
Rocuronium 10 mg/cc	0.6 mg/kg IV bolus	15 mg	▶ 1.5 cc

Fluid challenge: 480 ml NS or LR

Equipment

ETT	5.5–6 mm	Foley	10 Fr
ETT @ lip	17 cm	Chest tube	28 Fr
NG tube	12–14 Fr	Suction cath	10–14 Fr

Defibrillation: 48 J, 96 J, 96 J (2 J/kg, 4 J/kg, 4 J/kg)
Cardioversion: 12 J (0.5 J/kg)

30 kg		Heart rate	90
10 y		Respiratory rate	18–22
		Systolic BP	110 ± 15

Drug	Dose	Deliver (mg)	Deliver (cc)
Atropine	0.02 mg/kg	0.6 mg	▶ 6 cc
0.1 mg/cc	IV, IO, ET		
Dextrose 50%	0.5 g/kg	15 g	▶ 30 cc
0.5 g/cc	IV, IO		
Epinephrine	0.01 mg/kg	0.3 mg	▶ 3 cc
1:10,000	IV, IO		
Ketamine	1–2 mg/kg	30–60 mg	
	IV, IO		
Lorazepam	0.05–0.1 mg/kg	1.5–3 mg	▶ 0.75–1.5 cc
2 mg/cc	IV, IO		
Midazolam	0.05–0.1 mg/kg	1.5–3 mg	▶ 1.5–3 cc
1 mg/cc	IV, IO		
Rocuronium	0.6 mg/kg	18 mg	▶ 1.8 cc
10 mg/cc	IV bolus		

Fluid challenge: 600 ml NS or LR

Equipment

ETT	6–6.5 mm	Foley	12 Fr
ETT @ lip	18 cm	Chest tube	28–32 Fr
NG tube	14 Fr	Suction cath	14 Fr

Defibrillation: 60 J, 120 J, 120 J (2 J/kg, 4 J/kg, 4 J/kg)
Cardioversion: 15 J (0.5 J/kg)

40 kg		Heart rate	85
12 y		Respiratory rate	16–22
		Systolic BP	115 ± 20

Drug	Dose	Deliver (mg)	Deliver (cc)
Atropine 0.1 mg/cc	0.02 mg/kg IV, IO, ET	0.8 mg	► 8 cc
Dextrose 50% 0.5 g/cc	0.5 g/kg IV, IO	20 g	► 40 cc
Epinephrine 1:10,000	0.01 mg/kg IV, IO	0.4 mg	► 4 cc
Ketamine	1–2 mg/kg IV, IO	40–80 mg	
Lorazepam 2 mg/cc	0.05–0.1 mg/kg IV, IO	2–4 mg	► 1–2 cc
Midazolam 1 mg/cc	0.05–0.1 mg/kg IV, IO	2–4 mg	► 2–4 cc
Rocuronium 10 mg/cc	0.6 mg/kg IV bolus	24 mg	► 2.4 cc

Fluid challenge: 800 ml NS or LR

Equipment

ETT	6.5–7 mm	Foley	12 Fr
ETT @ lip	19 cm	Chest tube	28–32 Fr
NG tube	14 Fr	Suction cath	14 Fr

Defibrillation: 80 J, 160 J, 160 J (2 J/kg, 4 J/kg, 4 J/kg)
Cardioversion: 20 J (0.5 J/kg)

Instant Pediatric Medications

Age	3 mo	6 mo	9 mo	1 yr	18 mo	2 yr	3 yr	4 yr	5 yr	6 yr	8 yr	10 yr	12 yr
Wt kg	6	7	8.5	10	11	12	14	16	18	20	24	30	40
Atropine 0.1 mg/cc	0.12 mg	0.14 mg	0.17 mg	0.2 mg	0.22 mg	0.24 mg	0.28 mg	0.32 mg	0.36 mg	0.4 mg	0.48 mg	0.6 mg	0.8 mg
0.02 mg/Kg IV,IO, ET	1.2 cc	1.4 cc	1.7 cc	2 cc	2.2 cc	2.4 cc	2.8 cc	3.2 cc	3.6 cc	4 cc	4.8 cc	6 cc	8 cc
Epinephrine 1:10,000	0.06 mg	0.07 mg	0.08 mg	0.1 mg	0.11 mg	0.12 mg	0.14 mg	0.16 mg	0.18 mg	0.2 mg	0.24 mg	0.3 mg	0.4 mg
0.01 mg/Kg IV,IO, ET*	0.6 cc	0.7 cc	0.85 cc	1 cc	1.1 cc	1.2 cc	1.4 cc	1.6 cc	1.8 cc	2 cc	2.4 cc	3 cc	4 cc
Dextrose 50% 0.5 g/cc	**3 g	**3.5 g	**4.25 g	**5 g	**5.5 g	6 g	7 g	8 g	9 g	10 g	12 g	15 g	20 g
0.5 g/Kg IV,IO**	12cc	14 cc	17 cc	20 cc	22 cc	12 cc	14 cc	16 cc	18 cc	20 cc	24 cc	30 cc	40 cc
Sodium bicarbonate 8.4%***	6 mEq	7 mEq	8.5 mEq	10 mEq	11 mEq	12 mEq	14 mEq	16 mEq	18 mEq	20 mEq	24 mEq	30 mEq	40 mEq
1 mEq/Kg IV,IO	6 cc	7 cc	8.5 cc	10 cc	11 cc	12 cc	14 cc	16 cc	18 cc	20 cc	24 cc	30 cc	40 cc
Lidocaine 2% 20 mg/cc	6 mg	7 mg	8.5 mg	10 mg	11 mg	12 mg	14 mg	16 mg	18 mg	20 mg	24 mg	30 mg	40 mg
1 mg/Kg IV,IO	0.3 cc	0.35 cc	0.425 cc	0.5 cc	0.55 cc	0.6 cc	0.7 cc	0.8 cc	0.9 cc	1 cc	1.2 cc	1.5 cc	2 cc
Diazepam Valium® 5 mg/cc	1.5 mg	1.7 mg	2.12 mg	2.5 mg	2.7 mg	3 mg	3.5 mg	4 mg	4.5 mg	5 mg	6 mg	7.5 mg	10 mg
0.25 mg/Kg IV,IO, PR	0.3 cc	0.35 cc	0.42 cc	0.5 cc	0.55 cc	0.6 cc	0.7 cc	0.8 cc	0.9 cc	1 cc	1.2 cc	1.5 cc	2 cc
Lorazepam Ativan® 2 mg/cc	.3–.6 mg	.35–.7 mg	.42–.85 mg	.5–1 mg	.5–1.1 mg	.6–1.2 mg	.7–1.4 mg	.8–1.6 mg	.9–1.8 mg	1–2 mg	1.2–2.4 mg	1.5–3 mg	2–4 mg
0.05–0.1 mg/Kg IM,IV****	.15–.3 cc	.17–.35 cc	.21–.42 cc	.25–.5 cc	.25–.55 cc	.3–.6 cc	.35–.7 cc	.4–.8 cc	.45–.9 cc	.5–1 cc	.6–1.2 cc	.75–1.5 cc	1–2 cc

* Epinephrine: All endotracheal doses: 0.1 mg/kg (0.1 ml/kg of 1:1,000).
** Dilute D50 1:1 with sterile water to obtain D25 for infants.
*** Infants: Use 4.2% up to 3 months.
**** Dilute 1:1 for IV use.

Normal Vital Signs

Age	Prem	Term	3 mo	6 mo	9 mo	1 yr	18 mo	2 yr	3 yr	4 yr	5 yr	6 yr	8 yr	10 yr	12 yr
Wt Kg	1-2	3	6	7	8.5	10	11	12	14	16	18	20	24	30	40
Heart Rate	140	125	125	120	120	120	115	115	110	105	100	100	90	90	85
Respiration	<60	<60	36-48	24-36	24-32	22-30	22-28	22-28	20-26	20-26	20-24	20-24	18-22	18-22	16-22
Blood Press.	50-60	70	80±20	90±30	92±30	96±30	96±30	98±30	100±25	100±22	100±20	100±15	105±15	110±15	115±20
Equipment															
ETT tube mm*	2.5-3	3	3-3.5	3.5-4	3.5-4	4-4.5	4-4.5	4-4.5	4.5-5	4.5-5	5-5.5	5-5.5	5.5-6	6-6.5	6.5-7
ETT length cm	6+ kg	6+ kg	11	11	11	11	12	12	13	13	14	15	17	18	19
Laryngoscope Blade	0	1	1	1	1	1	1	1	2	2	2	2	2	2	3
Suction Cath Fr	8	8	8	8	8	8	8	8	10	10	10	10	10-14	14	14
NG tube Fr	5	5-8	8	8	8	8	8	10	10	10	10	12	12-14	14	14
Foley Fr		6	6	6-8	6-8	8	8	8	8-10	10	10	10	10	12	12
Chest tube Fr	10	12	12	12-16	16	20	20	20-24	20-24	24	24	28	28	28-32	28-32
IV Catheters	24	24	24-22	22	22	22-20	22-20	22-20	22-18	20-18	20-18	20-18	18	18	18-16
Fluid Challenge LR, NS 20 cc/kg 10 cc/kg neonate	15-20	30	120	140	170	200	220	240	280	320	360	400	480	600	800

*Have on hand 1 size larger and smaller

Common Antibiotics

Amoxicillin

Child: PO 20–50 mg/kg/24 h tid.

Ampicillin

Child, mild–moderate infections: IV, IM 100–200 mg/kg/24 h q 6 hours. PO 50–100 mg/kg/24 h q 6 hours. Max PO dose 2–3 g/24 h.

Azithromycin (Zithromax®)

Child > 6 mo, **otitis media or community-acquired pneumonia:** PO 10 mg/kg day 1 (not to exceed 500 mg), followed by 5 mg/kg/24 h q day (not to exceed 250 mg/24 h on days 2–5). **Pharyngitis,** child > 2 y: PO 12 mg/kg/24 h q day × 5 days (not to exceed 500 mg/24 h.)

Cefaclor (Ceclor®)

Infant and child: PO 20–40 mg/kg/24 h q 8 hours (max dose 2 g/24 h). Q 12-hour dosage interval optional in otitis media or pharyngitis.

Cefazolin (Ancef®, Kefzol®)

Infant > 1 mo and child: IV, IM 50–100 mg/kg/24 h q 8 hours (max dose 6 g/24 h).

Cefixime (Suprax®)

Infant and child: PO 8 mg/kg/24 h q12–24 hours (max dose 400 mg/24 h).

Cefoperazone (Cefobid®)

Infant and child: IV, IM 100–200 mg/kg/24 h q 8–12 hours.

Cefotaxime (Claforan®)

Infant and child < 50 kg: IV, IM 100–200 mg/kg/24 h q 6–8 hours. **Meningitis:** IV/IM 200 mg/kg/24 h q 6 hours (max dose 12 g/24 h).

Cefoxitin

Infant and child: IV, IM 80–160 mg/kg/24 h q 4–8 hours.

Cephalexin (Keflex®)

Infant and child: PO 25–100 mg/kg/24 h q 6 hours.

Ciprofloxacin (Cipro®)

Child: PO 20–30 mg/kg/24 h q 12 hours (max dose 1.5 g/24 h). IV 10–20 mg/kg/24 h q 12 hours (max dose 800 mg/24 h). **Cystic fibrosis:** PO 40 mg/kg/24 h q 12 hours (max dose 2 g/24 h). IV 30 mg/kg/24 h q 8 hours (max dose 1.2 g/24 h).

Dicloxacillin

Child < 40 kg **mild–moderate infections:** PO 12.5–25 mg/kg/24 h q 6 hours. **Severe infections:** PO 50–100 mg/kg/24 h q 6 hours.

Doxycycline (Vibramycin®)

Initial: < 45 kg: PO, IV 5 mg/kg/24 h bid × 1 day (max dose 200 mg/24 h). > 45 kg: PO, IV 100 mg bid × 1 day. **Maintenance:** < 45 kg: PO, IV 2.5–5 mg/kg/24 h q day bid. > 45 kg: PO, IV 100–200 mg/24 h q day bid.

Cardiology

Cardiology

Cardiology

Heart Sounds

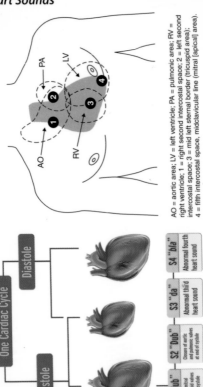

AO = aortic area; LV = left ventricle; PA = pulmonic area; RV = right ventricle; 1 = right second intercostal space; 2 = left second intercostal space; 3 = mid left sternal border (tricuspid area); 4 = fifth intercostal space, midclavicular line (mitral [apical] area).

One Cardiac Cycle

Systole

S1 "lub"
Closure of mitral and tricuspid valves at start of systole

S2 "Dub"
Closure of aortic and pulmonic valves at end of systole

Diastole

S3 "da"
Abnormal third heart sound

S4 "bla"
Abnormal fourth heart sound

S₁ Heard loudest at mitral and tricuspid areas. Associated with closure of mitral and tricuspid valves. Use diaphragm of stethoscope.

S₂ Heard loudest at aortic and pulmonic areas. Associated with closure of aortic and pulmonic valves. Use diaphragm of stethoscope.

S₃ Heard loudest at mitral area. "Ken-tuck-y" Associated with rapid ventricular filling. Use bell of stethoscope.

S₄ Heard loudest at mitral area. "Ten-nes-see" Associated with forceful atrial ejection into a distended ventricle. Use bell of stethoscope.

Cardiac Murmurs

Grade	Description
I	Barely audible.
II	Faint, clearly audible.
III	Moderately loud, no palpable thrill.
IV	Loud, palpable thrill likely.
V	Very loud, may be audible with stethoscope partly off chest. Palpable thrill likely.
VI	Very loud, may be audible with stethoscope off chest. Associated with palpable thrill.

Swan Ganz Waveforms

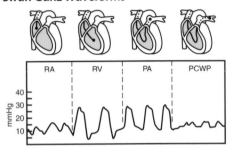

Cardioversion

Indications

Treatment of choice for tachyarrhythmias (SVT, VT, atrial fibrillation, atrial flutter) with evidence of cardiovascular compromise.

Precautions

Synchronized mode must be activated. If shock is present, intubation, ventilation with 100% oxygen, and vascular access are desirable, yet these therapies should not delay cardioversion. "Clear" before cardioversion.

Consider sedation if patient is conscious and time and condition allow.

Dose

Initial energy level: 0.5 J/kg. Second and subsequent energy levels: 1 J/kg.

If rhythm does not convert, reevaluate rhythm.

Defibrillation

Indications

First intervention for VF and pulseless VT.

Precautions

Do not delay shocks for VF or pulseless VT. Asystole should not be routinely shocked. "Clear" before defibrillation.

Dose

The initial energy level delivered is 2 J/kg followed by five cycles of CPR. If VF or pulseless VT continues, give a second shock at 4 J/kg. See the Pulseless Arrest algorithm on page 144 for more details.

Electrolyte Imbalance
Signs & Symptoms

Hypokalemia
Muscle weakness, hypotension, headache, dizziness, myocardial irritability. T wave flat, ST depressed.

Hyperkalemia
Bradycardia, asystole, muscle weakness, confusion. P wave flat, T wave peaked.

Hyponatremia
Hypotension, headache, tachycardia, lethargy, seizures, N/V, dry mucous membranes.

Hypernatremia
Hypertension, rales, tachycardia, oliguria, lethargy, irritability, tremors, flushed skin.

Hypocalcemia
Bronchospasm, muscle cramps, tremors, tetany, seizures, decreased cardiac output. QT interval long.

Hypercalcemia
Hypertension, anorexia, N/V, abdominal pain, headache, confusion, polydipsia, polyuria. QT interval short.

Hypomagnesemia
Dysrhythmias, enhanced digitalis effect, confusion, lethargy, coma, seizures, facial twitching. T wave flat, ST depressed, QT interval long.

Hypermagnesemia
Bradycardia, apnea, hypotension, muscle weakness, lethargy. T wave peaked.

Maintenance IV Fluids

First 10 kg body wt .... 100 ml/kg/day
Second 10 kg body wt .... 50 ml/kg/day
Each additional kg.................... 20 ml/kg/day

Example: A 23-kg child requires:
$(10 \times 100) + (10 \times 50) + (3 \times 20) = 1560$ ml/day

Fluid Resuscitation and Trauma

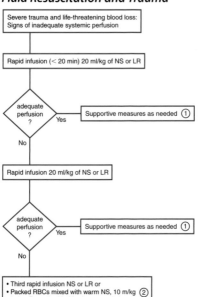

1 Consult Trauma Center.
2 Type and crossmatch blood emergently. Consider O-negative blood without
   crossmatch. Consult Trauma Center ASAP.

Neurology

Neurology

Reflexes

Babinski

Stroke sole of foot from heel to toes.
Abnormal response: Dorsiflexion and
fanning of toes.

Oculocephalic

Doll's eyes phenomenon should not be tested if
possibility of cervical spine injury exists.
Normal response: As head rotates, eyes lag, falling
in opposite direction, and slowly return to their
initial position.
Abnormal response: Eyes remain fixed as the head
is rotated.

Flexion

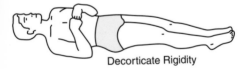

Decorticate Rigidity

Extension

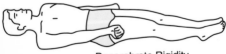

Decerebrate Rigidity

Dermatomes

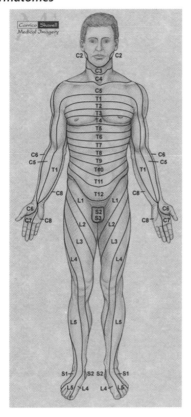

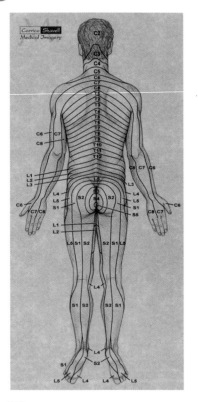

Pupil Gauge mm

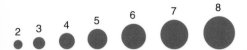

Glasgow Coma Scale

Infant/Toddler

Eye Opening		
Spontaneous	4
To Voice	3
To Pain	2
None	1

Best Verbal Response		
Smiles, Interacts	5
Consolable	4
Cries To Pain	3
Moans To Pain	2
None	1

Best Motor Response		
Normal Spont. Movement	6
Localizes Pain	5
Withdraws To Pain	4
Abnormal Flexion	3
Abnormal Extension	2
None	1

RR + SBP + GCS Points = RTS Total

Children/Adult

Eye Opening		
Spontaneous	4
To Voice	3
To Pain	2
None	1

Best Verbal Response		
Oriented	5
Confused	4
Inappropriate Words	3
Incomprehensible Words	2
None	1

Best Motor Response		
Obeys Command	6
Localizes Pain	5
Withdraws (Pain)	4
Flexion (Pain)	3
Extension (Pain)	2
None	1

Revised Trauma Score

Respiratory Rate		
10–29/min	4
>29/min	3
6–9/min	2
1–5/min	1
None	0

Systolic Blood Pressure		
>89 mm Hg	4
76–89 mm Hg	3
50–75 mm Hg	2
1–49 mm Hg	1
No Pulse	0

Total Glasgow Coma Scale Points		
13–15 = 4	RTS Subtotal _____
9–12 = 3	GCS _____
6–8 = 2	Points _____
4–5 = 1	RTS _____
3 = 0	Total _____

Appendix

Appendix

SODIUM BICARB .
QUINIDINE
PROCAINAMIDE
PHENYTOIN
NITROPRUSSIDE
NITROGLYCERINE
MORPHINE
MIDAZOLAM
METHYLPREDNISOLONE
MEPERIDINE
LORAZEPAM
LIDOCAINE
ISOPROTERENOL
INSULIN
HEPARIN
FUROSEMIDE
EPINEPHRINE
DOPAMINE
DOBUTAMINE
DIPHENHYDRAMINE
DIGOXIN
DIAZEPAM
AMRINONE
AMINOPHYLLINE

Drug Compatibility Matrix

C = Compatible at Y-Site
X = Incompatible at Y-Site
N = No/Not Enough
    Information

Aminophylline	—	C	N	C	C	X	C	X	C	C	X	X	C	C	C
Amrinone	C	—	N	N	N	C	C	N	N	N	N	N	C	N	X
Diazepam	X	N	—	N	N	X	X	N	N	N	N	C	N	C	X
Digoxin	C	N	N	—	N	N	N	C	N	N	C	N	N	N	X
Diphenhydramine	C	N	N	N	—	C	C	N	N	N	C	N	N	C	N
Dobutamine	X	C	X	N	C	—	C	N	X	N	C	C	C	N	X
Dopamine	C	C	X	N	C	C	—	N	N	N	N	C	C	N	X
Epinephrine	X	N	N	C	N	N	N	—	N	N	N	N	N	C	N
Furosemide	C	N	N	N	N	X	N	N	—	N	N	X	N	X	C
Heparin	C	N	N	N	N	N	N	N	N	—	X	C	N	N	C
Insulin	X	N	N	C	C	C	N	N	X	X	—	X	C	N	N
Isoproterenol	X	N	C	N	N	C	C	N	X	C	X	—	C	N	N
Lidocaine	C	C	N	N	N	C	C	N	N	N	C	C	—	C	X
Lorazepam	C	N	N	N	C	N	N	C	C	C	N	N	N	—	N

continues

Drug Compatibility Matrix, continued

| SODIUM BICARB. | PROCAINAMIDE | PROCAINAMIDE | PHENYTOIN | NITROPRUSSIDE | NITROGLYCERINE | MORPHINE | MIDAZOLAM | METHYLPREDNISOLONE | MEPERIDINE | LORAZEPAM | LIDOCAINE | ISOPROTERENOL | INSULIN | HEPARIN | FUROSEMIDE | EPINEPHRINE | DOPAMINE | DOBUTAMINE | DIPHENHYDRAMINE | DIGOXIN | AMRINONE | AMINOPHYLLINE |

C = Compatible at Y-Site
X = Incompatible at Y-Site
N = No/Not Enough Information

Meperidine	I	N	X	C	U	C	C	U	C	N	N	C	N	N	N	N	N	N	C	N	X	N	N	X
Methylprednisolone	C	N	N	N	N	N	N	C	U	N	C	N	C	N	N	N	N	N	N	N	N	|	N	N
Midazolam	X	N	N	N	N	N	N	N	N	N	N	N	C	N	N	N	N	N	X	N	N	N	N	N
Morphine	C	N	N	N	U	C	C	U	C	N	N	N	U	N	N	N	N	N	|	C	X	X	N	X
Nitroglycerine	C	N	N	N	N	N	C	U	C	N	N	N	N	N	N	N	N	N	N	N	N	|	N	N
Nitroprusside	N	X	N	N	N	N	N	N	N	C	N	N	N	N	N	N	N	|	N	X	X	N	N	N
Phenytoin	I	N	N	X	X	X	N	N	N	N	N	X	X	N	X	N	N	N	N	X	X	|	X	N
Procainamide	C	C	N	N	N	N	C	C	U	C	N	N	N	N	N	N	N	N	C	N	X	N	N	N
Quinidine	N	N	N	N	N	N	N	X	N	X	N	N	X	N	N	N	N	N	N	N	N	N	N	N
Sodium Bicarb.	C	X	X	N	N	N	U	N	X	N	N	X	N	N	N	X	N	X	N	X	N	N	X	N

Arterial Blood Gas Interpretation

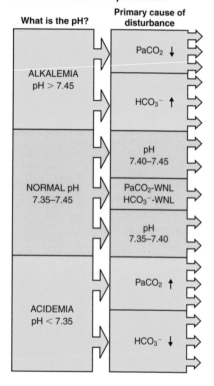

Has compensation taken place?	Term for acid-base condition	Current ventilatory status
HCO_3^--WNL	Uncompensated respiratory alkalosis	Alveolar hyperventilation a primary problem
HCO_3^- ↓	Partly compensated respiratory alkalosis	
HCO_3^- ↑ $PaCO_2$ ↓	Combined respiratory and metabolic alkalosis	
$PaCO_2$-WNL	Uncompensated metabolic alkalosis	Adequate alveolar ventilation for current demands
$PaCO_2$ ↑	Compensated metabolic alkalosis	Alveolar hypoventilation; normal ventilatory ability and reserve
HCO_3^- ↑ $PaCO_2$ ↑	Compensated respiratory alkalosis	
$PaCO_2$ ↓ HCO_3 ↓	Compensated respiratory alkalosis	Alveolar hypoventilation; a primary problem
Normal acid-base balance		Adequate alveolar ventilation
HCO_3^- ↓ $PaCO_2$ ↓	Compensated metabolic acidosis	Alveolar hyperventilation; ventilatory reserve available
$PaCO_2$ ↑ HCO_3^- ↑	Compensated respiratory acidosis	Chronic ventilatory insufficiency or failure
HCO_3^- ↑	Partly compensated respiratory acidosis	
HCO_3^--WNL	Uncompensated respiratory acidosis	Acute ventilatory failure
HCO_3^- ↓ $PaCO_2$ ↑	Combined respiratory and metabolic acidosis	
$PaCO_2$-WNL	Uncompensated metabolic acidosis	Adequate alveolar ventilation; inadequate ventilatory reserve
$PaCO_2$ ↓	Partly compensated metabolic acidosis	Alveolar hyperventilation; some ventilatory reserve

Blood Gases: Normal Values

	Arterial	Capillary	Venous
pH	7.35–7.45	7.35–7.45	7.31–7.41
PaO_2	80–100	40–60	35–40
$PaCO_2$	35–45	35–45	41–51
HCO_3	22–26	22–26	22–26
BE	± 2	± 2	± 2

Golden Rule #1
Calculating respiratory component of acid-base disorders: **An acute change in $PaCO_2$ of 10 torr is associated with an opposing increase or decrease in pH of 0.08 units.**

Blood Gases in Acidosis and Diabetes
Each 0.10 change in pH changes potassium 0.6 mmol/L in the opposite direction.

Example: If pH increases from 7.2 to 7.3, then potassium decreases from 3.4 to 2.8.

Rapid Sequence Intubation: Pediatric

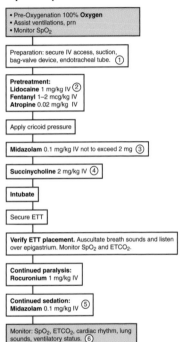

- Pre-Oxygenation 100% **Oxygen**
- Assist ventilations, prn
- Monitor SpO$_2$

Preparation: secure IV access, suction, bag-valve device, endotracheal tube. ①

Pretreatment:
Lidocaine 1 mg/kg IV ②
Fentanyl 1–2 mcg/kg IV
Atropine 0.02 mg/kg IV

Apply cricoid pressure

Midazolam 0.1 mg/kg IV not to exceed 2 mg ③

Succinylcholine 2 mg/kg IV ④

Intubate

Secure ETT

Verify ETT placement. Auscultate breath sounds and listen over epigastrium. Monitor SpO$_2$ and ETCO$_2$.

Continued paralysis:
Rocuronium 1 mg/kg IV

Continued sedation:
Midazolam 0.1 mg/kg IV ⑤

Monitor: SpO$_2$, ETCO$_2$, cardiac rhythm, lung sounds, ventilatory status. ⑥

1 ETT: have on hand, one size smaller and one size larger as you prepare to intubate.
2 Administer **lidocaine** in the presence of head injury.
3 May use etomidate or ketamine.
4 Succinylcholine is contraindicated if family history of **malignant hyperthermia** exists; in cases of penetrating eye injury, hyperkalemia and severe burn and crush injuries that are 2–5 days old. The onset of **succinylcholine** is 30–60 seconds, duration is 8–10 minutes.
5 Consider pain control measures. Paralytics and sedatives do not alter pain.
6 **Keep the patient warm.** Paralyzed patients lose much of their ability to generate body heat.

Burn Management

Area	Age (y)			
	0–1	1–4	4–9	10–15
Head	19	17	13	10
Neck	2	2	2	2
Trunk	13	13	13	13
Buttock, R/L	2.5	2.5	2.5	2.5
Genitalia	1	1	1	1
Upper arm, R/L	4	4	4	4
Lower arm, R/L	3	3	3	3
Hand, R/L	2.5	2.5	2.5	2.5
Thigh, R/L	5.5	6.5	8.5	8.5
Leg, R/L	5	5	5	6
Foot, R/L	3.5	3.5	3.5	3.5

Lund-Browder chart: % BSA estimates according to age.

Major Burn

- 25% of the body surface or greater
- Significant involvement of hand, face, joints, feet, or perineum
- Electrical injury
- Inhalation injury
- Concomitant injury
- Severe preexisting medical problems

Major burns should be treated at a burn unit.

American Burn Association

Parkland Formula

First 24 hours: If less than 30% BSA has second- or third-degree burns, give lactated Ringer's (LR) 3 ml/kg × % BSA burned. If more than 30% BSA, give LR 4 ml/kg × % BSA. Give half of this total over the first 8 hours, calculated from time of injury. Give the balance over the next 16 hours.

Second day: Fluid requirements average 50% to 75% of first day's requirement.

Consider adding colloid after 18–24 hours (1 g/kg/day of albumin) to maintain serum albumin greater than 2 g/100 ml.

Withhold potassium for the first 48 hours.

Galveston Formula

First 24 hours: Give 5000 ml/m² of burned area plus 2000 ml/m² of total BSA (maintenance fluids) over the first 24 hours; give one-half over the first 8 hours calculated from time of injury. For children older than 1 year, use LR + 12.5 g 25% albumin/liter. For infants younger than 1 year, prepare a 1-liter solution of 930 ml of 1/3 NS, 20 ml sodium bicarbonate (1 mEq/ml), and 50 ml of 25% albumin.

Second day: Give 3750 ml/m² of burned area/24 h plus 1500 ml/m² of total BSA/24 h (maintenance fluids). Since sodium requirements after the first 24 hours are less, use D5 1/3NS with 20–30 mEq/L of potassium phosphate.

Hypothermia

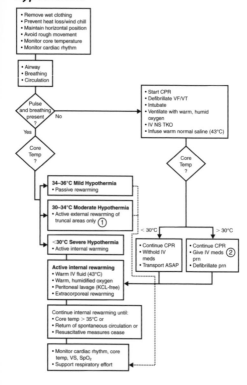

1   Methods include warm water bottles, heating pads, radiant heat sources, and warming beds.

2   Give IV medications at longer than standard intervals.

Physiology of Hypothermia

	°C	°F	Characteristics
M	**37**	98.6	Normal temperature.
I	**36**	96.8	Increase in basal metabolic rate.
L	**35**	95	Maximum shivering.
D	**34**	93.2	Amnesia, normal BP.
	33	91.4	Ataxia develops.
M	**32**	89.6	Stupor, 25% decrease in O_2 consumption.
O	**31**	87.8	Shivering stops.
D	**30**	86	Atrial fibrillation and other dysrhythmias. Pulse, cardiac output 66% normal.
E			
R			
A			
T	**29**	85.2	Progressive decrease in LOC, pulse, respirations. Pupils dilate.
E			
	28	82.4	VF susceptibility, 50% decrease in O_2 consumption and pulse.
	27	80.6	Losing reflexes and voluntary motion.
S	**26**	78.8	No reflexes or response to pain.
E	**25**	77	Cerebral blood flow 33% normal, cardiac output 45% normal.
V			
E	**24**	75.2	Significant hypotension.
R	**23**	73.4	No corneal reflexes.
E	**22**	71.6	75% decrease in O_2 consumption. Maximum risk of VF.
	19	66.2	Flat EEG.
	18	64.4	Asystole develops.

Source: Danzl DF: Accidental Hypothermia. *Emergency Medicine: Current Concepts in Clinical Practice,* edited by Rosen P, Baker GR, et al. C. V. Mosby, 1983.

Metric Conversions

Volume
1 teaspoon = 5 ml
1 tablespoon = 15 ml
1 fluid oz = 30 ml
1 cup = 240 ml
1 pint = 473 ml
1 quart = 946 ml

Weight
1 g = 1,000 mg
1 mg = 1,000 mcg
1 kg = 2.2 lbs

Pressure
1 mmHg = 1.36 cmH$_2$O
1 cmH$_2$O = 0.73 mmHg

Temp		Weight	
C°	F°	Kg	lbs
40.6	105.1	125	275
40.4	104.7	120	264
40.2	104.3	115	253
40.0	104.0	110	242
39.8	103.7	105	231
39.6	103.3	100	220
39.4	102.9	95	209
39.2	102.6	90	198
39.0	102.2	85	187
38.8	101.8	80	176
38.6	101.5	75	165
38.4	101.2	70	154
38.2	100.8	65	143
38.0	100.4	60	132
37.8	100.1	55	121
37.6	99.7	50	110
37.4	99.3	45	99
37.2	99.0	40	88
37.0	**98.6**	35	77
36.0	96.8	30	66
35.0	95.0	25	55
34.0	93.2	20	44
33.0	91.4	15	33
32.0	89.6	10	22
31.0	87.8	7	15
30.0	86.0	5	11
29.0	85.2	3.5	7.5
28.0	82.4	1.5	3.0
27.0	80.6	1	2.2

Body Surface Area

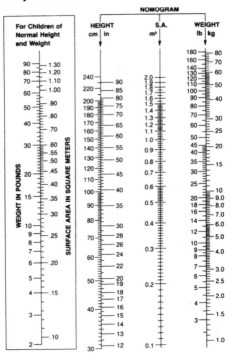

Nomogram for estimating surface area in children. From Behrman RE, et al., eds. *Nelson Textbook of Pediatrics* (16th ed.). Philadelphia: WB Saunders, 2000.

Normal Laboratory Values
Chemistry

Sodium	136–145 mmol/L
Potassium	3.5–5.5 mmol/L
Chloride	95–107 mmol/L
CO_2	20–28 mmol/L
BUN	7–18 mg/dl
Creatinine	0.7–1.2 mg/dl
Glucose	
premature	20–65 mg/dl
term	20–110 mg/dl
1 wk–16 yr	60–105 mg/dl
Calcium	8.5–10.6 mg/dl
Magnesium	1.3–2.1 mEq/L
Osmolality	285–295 mOsm/kg
Amylase	0–88 U/L

Bilirubin total

0–1 day	preterm	< 8 mg/dl
	term	< 6 mg/dl
1–2 days	preterm	<12 mg/dl
	term	< 8 mg/dl
3–7 days	preterm	< 16 mg/dl
	term	< 12 mg/dl
7–30 days	preterm	< 12 mg/dl
	term	< 7 mg/dl
thereafter	preterm	< 2 mg/dl
	term	< 1 mg/dl

Normal laboratory values vary from lab to lab.

Coagulation

Prothrombin Time (PT)

preterm	12–21 seconds
term	13–20 seconds
child	12–14 seconds

Time Activated (aPTT)

preterm	70 seconds
term	45–65 seconds
child	30–45 seconds

Fibrinogen   200–400 mg/dl

INR

1–5 yr	0.96–1.04
6–10 yr	0.91–1.11
11–16 yr	0.93–1.10

Hematology

Age	Hgb g%	Hct %	WBC/mm³ x 1000	Platelets 10³/mm³
term	16.5	51	18.1	290
1–3 days	18.5	56	18.9	192
2 wk	16.6	53	11.4	252
1 mo	13.9	44	10.8	
2 mo	11.2	35		
6 mo	12.6	36	11.9	
6 mo–2 yr	12.0	36	10.6	150–350
2–6 yr	12.5	37	8.5	150–350
6–12 yr	13.5	40	8.1	150–350
12–18 yr	14.5	43	7.8	150–350

Drug Toxicity

Drug	Half Life Hours	Elimination % Renal	Elimination % Hepatic	Therapeutic Blood Level mg/L	Toxicity: Signs & Symptoms
Acetaminophen Tylenol®	2	0	100	5–20	GI symptoms, malaise, pallor, diaphoresis. Elevated bilirubin, PTT, hepatic enzymes.
Amitriptyline	16	2	98	0.12–0.25	Drowsiness, hypotension, tachycardia, coma, conduction delays, CHF, seizures, hypothermia.
Digoxin	42	70	30	0.5–2 mcg/L	Anorexia, N/V, changes in visual acuity and color perception. PVCs, VT, junctional tachycardia, AV block, PSVT with block, sinus arrest, hyperkalemia.
Lidocaine	1.8	5	9	1.5–5	Lightheadedness, confusion, seizures, paresthesias, AV block, asystole.
Nitroprusside Nitropress®	very brief	0	100		Profound hypotension. Cyanide toxicity: dyspnea, headache, coma, V, dizziness, ataxia, dilated pupils, absent reflexes, pink color, distant heart tones. Thiocyanate blood levels should not exceed 10 mg/dl.
Pentobarbital Nembutal®	15–48	86	14	1–4	Hypotension, laryngospasm, hypothermia, pulmonary edema, renal failure.

Phenytoin Dilantin®	24	2	98	10–20	Lateral gaze nystagmus, ataxia, confusion, lethargy, paradoxical increase in seizures, dysrhythmias, hypotension.
Procainamide Pronestyl®	2–5	50	50	4–10	Prolonged QRS and QT. Impaired AV conduction, VF, hypotension.
Salicylate Aspirin	3–6†† 15–30†	50	100	20–250	Tinnitus, dizziness, headache, confusion, N/V, acid base imbalances, hyperthermia.
Theophylline	6–10	0	100	10–20	N/V, dysrhythmias, seizures.

†† Acute administration   † Chronic administration

Cerebrospinal Fluid: Differential Diagnosis

Condition	Color	Pressure (mm H_2O)	Protein (mg/100 ml)	Glucose (mg/100 ml)	Cells (no. per mm³)
Adult normal values	Clear	70–180	15–45	45–80	0–5 lymphs
Newborn normal values	Clear	70–180	20–120	2/3 serum	40–60 lymphs
Viral infection	Clear or opalescent	Normal or slight increase	Normal or slight increase	Normal	10–500 lymphs; poly early
Bacterial infection	Yellow; may clot	Increased	50–1500	< 20	25–10,000 polys
Subarachnoid hemorrhage	Bloody	Usually increased	Increased	Normal	WBC/RBC ratio same as blood

Blood Products

	Time	Storage	Infusion	Note
Packed RBCs	1 hr to type & cross-match		Infuse no faster than 2–3 ml/kg/hr	Type and crossmatch where possible. Watch for s/sx of reaction.
Fresh Frozen Plasma	30 min to thaw, use within 24 hr		Infuse over 2–4 hr Dose: 10–15 ml/kg, repeat as needed	Contains all clotting factors except platelets. Watch for s/sx of reaction.
Platelets	Use within 4 hr of pooling	Continuously agitate, room temperature	Infuse rapidly: 1–2 ml/min	10 ml/kg will increase platelet count by approximately 50,000/mm^3.
Cryoprecipitate	20 min to thaw, use within 4 hr	Obtain just prior to infusion	Dose: 1 bag/5 kg	Useful in factor VIII, vWF, and fibrinogen deficiency in context of active bleeding. 1 unit of cryoprecipitate/10 kg body wt. Increases fibrinogen by approx. 50 mg/dl.

*Dispensing pin available to allow 24 hr use.

Apgar Score and Newborn Vital Signs

Term Newborn Vital Signs (first 12 hours of life)

Heart rate (awake)	100 to 180 bpm
Respiratory rate	30 to 60 breaths/min
Systolic blood pressure	39 to 59 mmHg
Diastolic blood pressure	16 to 36 mmHg

Apgar Score			
Sign	0	1	2
Heart rate (bpm)	Absent	Slow (< 100)	≥ 100
Respirations	Absent	Slow, irregular	Good, crying
Muscle tone	Limp	Some flexion	Active motion
Reflex irritability (catheter in nares, tactile stimulation)	No response	Grimace	Cough, sneeze, cry
Color	Blue or pale	Pink body with blue extremities	Completely pink

Recommended Childhood and Adolescent Immunization Schedule · UNITED STATES · 2006

Vaccine ▼ Age ▶	Birth	1 month	2 months	4 months	6 months	12 months	15 months	18 months	24 months	4-6 years	11-12 years	13-14 years	15 years	16-18 years
Hepatitis B[1]	HepB	HepB		HepB[1]		HepB					HepB Series			
Diphtheria, Tetanus, Pertussis[2]			DTaP	DTaP	DTaP		DTaP			DTaP	Tdap	Tdap	Tdap	
Haemophilus influenzae type b[3]			Hib	Hib	Hib[3]	Hib								
Inactivated Poliovirus			IPV	IPV		IPV				IPV				
Measles, Mumps, Rubella[4]						MMR				MMR	MMR			
Varicella[5]						Varicella					Varicella			
Meningococcal[6]									MPSV4		MCV4	MCV4		MCV4
Pneumococcal[7]			PCV	PCV	PCV	PCV			PCV		PPV			
Influenza[8]					Influenza (Yearly)				Influenza (Yearly)		Influenza (Yearly)			
Hepatitis A[9]									HepA Series					

This schedule indicates the recommended ages for routine administration of currently licensed childhood vaccines, as of December 1, 2005, for children through age 18 years. Any dose not given at the recommended age should be administered at any subsequent visit when indicated and feasible. ▇ Indicates age groups that warrant special effort to administer those vaccines not previously administered. Additional vaccines may be licensed and recommended during the year. Licensed combination vaccines may be used whenever any components of the combination are indicated and other components of the vaccine are not contraindicated and if approved by the Food and Drug Administration for that dose of the series. Providers should consult the respective ACIP statement for detailed recommendations. Clinically significant adverse events that follow immunization should be reported to the Vaccine Adverse Event Reporting System (VAERS). Guidance about how to obtain and complete a VAERS form is available at www.vaers.hhs.gov or by telephone, 800-822-7967.

▇ Range of recommended ages
▇ 11–12-year-old assessment
▇ Catch-up immunization

FOOTNOTES ON REVERSE SIDE

DEPARTMENT OF HEALTH AND HUMAN SERVICES
CENTERS FOR DISEASE CONTROL AND PREVENTION
SAFER · HEALTHIER · PEOPLE."

The Childhood and Adolescent Immunization Schedule is approved by:
Advisory Committee on Immunization Practices www.cdc.gov/nip/acip
American Academy of Pediatrics www.aap.org
American Academy of Family Physicians www.aafp.org

More information regarding vaccine administration can be obtained at www.cdc.gov/nip or the CDC-INFO contact center
800-CDC-INFO
(ENGLISH & ESPAÑOL) – 24/7
[800-232-4636]

Keep track of your child's immunizations
CDC Childhood Immunization Scheduler www.cdc.gov/nip/kidstuff/scheduler.htm

FOOTNOTES

1. Hepatitis B vaccine (HepB): *AT BIRTH:* All newborns should receive monovalent HepB soon after birth and before hospital discharge. Infants born to mothers who are HBsAg-positive should receive HepB and 0.5 mL of hepatitis B immune globulin (HBIG) within 12 hours of birth. Infants born to mothers whose HBsAg status is unknown should receive HepB within 12 hours of birth. The mother should have her blood drawn as soon as possible to determine her HBsAg status; if HBsAg-positive, the infant should receive HBIG as soon as possible (no later than age 1 week). *For infants born to HBsAg-negative mothers,* the birth dose can be delayed in rare circumstances but only if a physician's order to withhold the vaccine and a copy of the mother's original HBsAg-negative laboratory report are documented in the infant's medical record. *FOLLOWING THE BIRTH DOSE:* The HepB series should be completed with either monovalent HepB or a combination vaccine containing HepB. The second dose should be administered at age 1–2 months. The final dose should be administered at age ≥24 weeks. It is permissible to administer 4 doses of HepB (e.g., when combination vaccines are administered after the birth dose); however, if monovalent HepB is used, a dose at age 4 months is not needed. Infants born to HBsAg-positive mothers should be tested for HBsAg and antibody to HBsAg after completion of the HepB series at age 9–18 months (generally at the next well-child visit after completion of the vaccine series).

2. Diphtheria and tetanus toxoids and acellular pertussis vaccine (DTaP). The fourth dose of DTaP may be administered as early as age 12 months, provided 6 months have elapsed since the third dose and the child is unlikely to return at age 15–18 months. The final dose in the series should be administered at age 4–6 years.

Tetanus and diphtheria toxoids and acellular pertussis vaccine (Tdap – adolescent preparation) is recommended at age 11–12 years for those who have completed the recommended childhood DTP/DTaP vaccination series and have not received a Td booster dose. Adolescents aged 13–18 years who missed the 11–12 year Td/Tdap booster dose should also receive a single dose of Tdap if they have completed the recommended childhood DTP/DTaP vaccination series. Refer to the ACIP statement **tetanus and diphtheria toxoids (Td)** are recommended every 10 years.

3. Haemophilus influenzae type b conjugate vaccine (Hib). Three Hib conjugate vaccines are licensed for infant use. If PRP-OMP (PedvaxHIB® or COMVAX® [Merck]) is administered at ages 2 and 4 months, a dose at age 6 months is not required. DTaP/Hib combination products should not be used for primary immunization in infants at ages 2, 4, or 6 months but can be used as boosters after any Hib vaccine. The final dose in the series should be administered at age ≥12 months.

4. Measles, mumps, and rubella vaccine (MMR). The second dose of MMR is recommended routinely at age 4–6 years but may be administered during any visit, provided at least 4 weeks have elapsed since the first dose and both doses are administered beginning at or after age 12 months. Children who have not previously received the second dose should complete the schedule by age 11–12 years.

5. Varicella vaccine. Varicella vaccine is recommended at any visit at or after age 12 months for susceptible children (i.e., those who lack a reliable history of chickenpox). Susceptible persons aged ≥13 years should receive 2 doses administered at least 4 weeks apart.

6. Meningococcal conjugate vaccine (MCV4). Meningococcal conjugate vaccine (MCV4) should be given to all children at the 11–12 year old visit as well as to unvaccinated adolescents at high school entry (age 15 years). Other adolescents who wish to decrease their risk for meningococcal disease may also be vaccinated. All college freshmen living in dormitories should also be vaccinated, preferably with MCV4, although **meningococcal polysaccharide vaccine (MPSV4)** is an acceptable alternative. Vaccination with MCV4 is recommended for children and adolescents aged ≥2 years with terminal complement deficiencies or anatomic or functional asplenia and for certain other high-risk groups [see *MMWR* 2005;54 (RR-7):1-21]; use MPSV4 for children aged 2–10 years and MCV4 for older children, although MPSV4 is an acceptable alternative.

7. Pneumococcal vaccine. The heptavalent pneumococcal conjugate vaccine (PCV) is recommended for all children ages 2–23 months and for certain children aged 24–59 months. The final dose in the series should be administered at age ≥12 months. **Pneumococcal polysaccharide vaccine (PPV)** is recommended in addition to PCV for certain high-risk groups. See *MMWR* 2000; 49(RR-9):1-35.

8. Influenza vaccine. Influenza vaccine is recommended annually for children aged ≥6 months with certain risk factors (including, but not limited to, asthma, cardiac disease, sickle cell disease, human immunodeficiency virus [HIV], diabetes, and conditions that can compromise respiratory function or handling of respiratory secretions or that can increase the risk for aspiration), healthcare workers, and other persons (including household members) in close contact with persons in groups at high risk [see *MMWR* 2005;54(RR-8):1-55]. In addition, healthy children aged 6–23 months and close contacts of healthy children aged 0–23 months are recommended to receive influenza vaccine because children in this age group are at substantially increased risk for influenza-related hospitalizations. For healthy persons aged 5–49 years, the intranasally administered, live, attenuated influenza vaccine (LAIV) is an acceptable alternative to the intramuscular trivalent inactivated influenza vaccine (TIV). See [*MMWR* 2005;54(RR-8):1-55. Children receiving TIV should be given a dosage appropriate for their age (0.25 mL if aged 6–35 months or 0.5 mL if aged ≥3 years). Children aged ≤8 years who are receiving influenza vaccine for the first time should receive 2 doses (separated by at least 4 weeks for TIV and at least 6 weeks for LAIV).

9. Hepatitis A vaccine (HepA). HepA is recommended for all children at 1 year of age (i.e., 12–23 months). The 2 doses in the series should be administered at least 6 months apart. States, counties, and communities with existing HepA vaccination programs for children aged 2–18 years are encouraged to maintain these programs. In these areas, new efforts focused on routine vaccination of 1-year-old children should enhance, not replace, ongoing programs directed at a broader population of children. HepA is also recommended for certain high-risk groups [see *MMWR* 1999; 48(RR-12):1-37].

Organ Donation

When the patient dies…

1. Recognize the patient as potential organ and/or tissue donor.
2. Continue your role as patient and family advocate, and champion their right to consider donation.
3. Before offering the option of donation to the family, consult your local organ procurement organization for specific eligibility.
4. Separate the discussion regarding the pronouncement of death from that of donation. Allow the family time to acknowledge that death has occurred before discussing donation.
5. When offering the option of donation:
   - Identify the next of kin.
   - Use short concise sentences.
   - Ask the family, "Do you know if [name] ever signed a donor card?" or "Did you ever discuss donation with [name]?"
   - Use the term "dead." Euphemisms like "passed on" may be confusing.
   - Use the term "recovery" of organs. Many families find the term "harvest" offensive.

Source: U.S. Department of Health & Human Services

For the name & phone number of your local recovery agency call **1-800-292-9537**.

Numeric Pain Scale

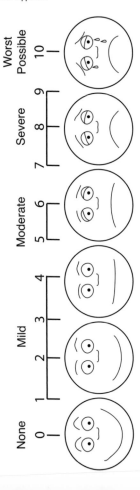

Generic and Brand Name Index

Generic name is indicated by **BOLD** upper case.
Brand name is indicated by blue.
Classification(s) or indication(s) follow.

ABACAVIR Ziagen anti-infective, HIV
Abilify **ARIPIPRAZOLE** schizophrenia
Abitrate **CLOFIBRATE** anti-hyperlipidemic
Abitrexate **METHOTREXATE** oncology
ACARBOSE Precose hypoglycemic
Accolate **ZAFIRLUKAST** inhibits bronchospasm
AccuNeb **ALBUTEROL** bronchodilator
Accupril **QUINAPRIL** antihypertensive
Accuretic **QUINAPRIL/THIAZIDE** antihypertensive
Accutane **ISOTRETINOIN** antiacne agent
ACEBUTOLOL Sectral antihypertensive
Aceon **PERINDOPRIL** antihypertensive
Acetadote **ACETYLCYSTEINE** acetaminophen OD
ACETAMINOPHEN Tylenol antipyretic
ACETAZOLAMIDE Diamox, Dazamide diuretic,
    anticonvulsant
ACETOHEXAMIDE Dymelor diabetes
ACETOHYDROXAMIC ACID Lithostat UTI
ACETYLCYSTEINE Mucomyst antidote for
    acetaminophen OD
Achromycin **TETRACYCLINE** antibiotic
AcipHex **RABEPRAZOLE** gastric acid inhibitor
ACITRETIN Soriatane severe psoriasis
Aclovate **ALCLOMETASONE** steroid
Acova **ARGATROBAN** anticoagulant
Actigall **URSODIOL** gallstones
Activase **ALTEPLASE** TPA thrombolytic
Activella **ESTRADIOL** hormone, menopause
Actonel **RISEDRONATE** Paget's disease, osteoporosis
Actos **PIOGLITAZONE** type II diabetes
Actron **KETOPROFEN** NSAID

Acular Ophthalmic **KETOROLAC** NSAID

Adalat **NIFEDIPINE** calcium channel blocker

ADALIMUMAB Humira rheumatoid arthritis

ADAPALENE Differin acne

Adapin **DOXEPIN** tricyclic antidepressant

Adderall **DEXTROAMPHETAMINE &
AMPHETAMINE** ADHD

Adenocard **ADENOSINE** antiarrhythmic

ADENOSINE Adenocard antiarrhythmic

Adipex-P **PHENTERMINE HCL** appetite suppressant

Adipost **PHENDIMETRAZINE** appetite suppressant

Adriamycin **DOXORUBICIN** antibiotic, oncology

Adrucil **FLUOROURACIL** oncology

Adsorbocarpine **PILOCARPINE** antiglaucoma

Advair DisKus **FLUTICASONE & SALMETEROL**
steroid

Advil **IBUPROFEN** NSAID

Aerobid **FLUNISOLIDE** steroid

Aerolate **THEOPHYLLINE** bronchodilator

Aerosporin **POLYMYXIN B** antibiotic

Aggrastat **TIROFIBAN** unstable angina

Agrylin **ANAGRELIDE** platelet aggregation inhibitor

Akineton **BIPERIDEN** anti-Parkinson's

ALBUTEROL AccuNeb, Proventil, Ventolin, Volmax
bronchodilator

Aldactazide **HCTZ & PIRONOLACTONE** diuretic

Aldactone **SPIRONOLACTONE** diuretic

Aldara **IMIQUIMOB** treat genital warts

Aldomet **METHYLDOPA** antihypertensive

ALENDRONATE Fosamax osteoporosis

Aleve **NAPROXEN** NSAID

ALFUZOSIN Uroxatral muscle relaxer

ALITRETINOIN Panretin oncology

Alkeran **MELPHALAN** anticancer agent

Allegra **FEXOFENADINE** antihistamine

Aller-Chlor **CHLORPHENIRAMINE** antihistamine

ALLOPURINOL Aloprim, Zyloprim anti-gout
ALMOTRIPTAN Axert treat migraine
Aloprim **ALLOPURINOL** anti-gout
Alora Transdermal **ESTRADIOL** estrogen
ALOSETRON Lotronex Crohn's disease
Aloxi **PALONOSETRON** antiemetic
ALPRAZOLAM Xanax sedative benzodiazepine
Altace **RAMIPRIL** ACE inhibitor antihypertensive
ALPROSTADIL Caverject, Edex erectile dysfunction
ALTEPLASE Activase TPA thrombolytic
ALTRERAMINE Hexalen oncology
Alupent **METAPROTERENOL** bronchodilator
AMANTADINE Symmetrel, Symadine anti-Parkinson's
Amaryl **GLIMEPIRIDE** diabetes
AMBENONIUM Mytelase myasthenia gravis
Ambien **ZOLPIDEM** insomnia
Amcort **TRIAMCINOLONE** steroid
Amerge **NARATRIPTAN** cluster headache in adults
AMIFOSTINE Ethyol oncology
AMIKACIN Amikin antibiotic
Amikin **AMIKACIN** antibiotic
Amiloride **MIDAMOR** diuretic
AMINOPHYLLINE Somophyllin bronchodilator
AMIODARONE Cordarone refractory VTach
AMITRIPTYLINE Vanatrip tricyclic antidepressant
AMLODIPINE Norvasc calcium channel blocker
AMLODIPINE & BENAZEPRIL Lotrel antihypertensive
AMOXAPINE Asendin tricyclic antidepressant
AMOXICILLIN Amoxicot, Amoxil, Trimox antibiotic
Amoxicot **AMOXICILLIN** antibiotic
Amoxil **AMOXICILLIN** antibiotic
AMPHETAMINE CNS stimulant
AMPICILLIN Marcillin, Omnipen, Polycillin antibiotic
AMRINONE Inocor inotropic agent
Anafranil **CLOMIPRAMINE** tricyclic antidepressant
ANAGRELIDE Agrylin essential thrombocythemia

ANAKINRA Kineret anti-rheumatic
Anaprox **NAPROXEN** NSAID
Anaspaz **HYOSCYAMINE** stomach disorders
ANASTROZOLE Arimidex oncology
Ancef **CEFAZOLIN** antibiotic
Ancobon **FLUCYTOSINE** antifungal
Android-F **FLUOXYMESTERONE** oncology
Anectine **SUCCINYLCHOLINE** neuromuscular blocker
Anergan **PROMETHAZINE** antiemetic
Anexsia **ACETAMINOPHEN & HYDROCODONE**
Angiomax **BIVALIRUDIN** anticoagulant
ANISTREPLASE Eminase thrombolytic
Ansaid **FLURBIPROFEN** NSAID
Antabuse **DISULFIRAM** alcohol abuse deterrent
ANTIPYRINE & BENZOCAINE Auralgan otic analgesic
Antivert **MECLIZINE** antiemetic; vertigo
Anxanil **HYDROXYZINE** sedative
Anzemet **DOLASETRON** antiemetic
Apo-Metformin **METFORMIN** type II diabetes
Apresoline **HYDRALAZINE** diuretic antihypertensive
APROTININ Trasylol blood loss during repeat CABG
AquaMEPHYTOIN **PHYTONADIONE** vitamin K
Aquatensen **METHYCLOTHIAZIDE** diuretic
Aquazide **HYDROCHLOROTHIAZIDE** diuretic
Arava **LEFLUNOMIDE** anti-inflammatory
Aramine **METARAMINOL** vasopressor
Aredia **PAMIDRONATE** electrolyte modifier
ARGATROBAN Acova anticoagulant
Aricept **DONEPEZIL** Alzheimer's disease
Arimidex **ANASTROZOLE** oncology
ARIPIPRAZOLE Abilify schizophrenia
Aromasin **EXEMESTANE** oncology
ARSENIC Trisenox leukemia
Artane **TRIHEXYPHENIDYL** anti-Parkinson's
Arthropan **CHOLINE SALICYLATE** analgesic
ASA ASPIRIN analgesic, antipyretic

Asacol **MESALAMINE** Crohn's disease

Asendin **AMOXAPINE** tricyclic antidepressant

Asminyl **DYPHYLLINE** bronchodilator

ASPARAGINASE Elspar oncology

A-Spas **HYOSCYAMINE** stomach disorders

Atacand **CANDESARTAN CILEXETIL** hypertension

Atapryl **SELEGILINE** MAO inhibitor, anti-Parkinson's

Atarax **HYDROXYZINE** sedative hypnotic

ATAZANAVIR Reyataz HIV

ATENOLOL Tenormin antihypertensive, β-blocker

Ativan **LORAZEPAM** benzodiazepine, antianxiety

ATOMOXETINE Strattera attention deficit disorder

ATORVASTATIN Lipitor elevated total cholesterol

ATOVAQUONE Mepron antibiotic

ATRACURIUM Tracrium neuromuscular blocking
agent

Atretol **CARBAMAZEPINE** anticonvulsant

Atromid-S **CLOFIBRATE** lipid lowering agent

Atrovent **IPRATROPIUM** bronchodilator

Augmentin **AMOXICILLIN & CLAVULANATE**
antibiotic

Auralgan **ANTIPYRINE & BENZOCAINE** otic analgesic

AURANOFIN Ridaura anti-inflammatory

Avandamet **ROSIGLITAZONE & METFORMIN**
diabetes

Avandia **ROSIGLITAZONE** diabetes

Avapro **IRBESARTAN** hypertension

Avastin **BEVACIZUMAB** oncology

Avelox **MOXIFLOXACIN** antibiotic

Aventyl **NORTRIPTYLINE** tricyclic antidepressant

Avita **TRETINOIN** acne

Axert **ALMOTRIPTAN** treat migraine

Axid **NIZATIDINE** antiulcer

Azactam **AZTREONAM** antibiotic

AZATHIOPRINE Imuran immunosuppressant

AZITHROMYCIN Zithromax antibiotic

Azmacort **TRIAMCINOLONE** steroid, asthma
AZT antiviral
AZTREONAM Azactam antibiotic
Azulfidine **SULFASALAZINE** antibiotic

BACAMPICILLIN Spectrobid antibiotic
Baci-IM **BACITRACIN** antibiotic
BACITRACIN Baci-IM antibiotic
BACLOFEN Lioresal skeletal muscle relaxant
Bactocill **OXACILLIN** antibiotic
Bactrim **TRIMETHOPRIM & SULFAMETOXAZOLE**
    antibiotic
Bactroban **MUPIROCIN** antibiotic
BALSALAZIDE Colazal anti-inflammatory
Baycol **CERIVASTATIN** elevated cholesterol
Becloforte **BECLOMETHASONE** asthma
BECLOMETHASONE Beconase, Vancenase
    glucocorticoid
Beclovent **BETACLOMETHASONE** asthma
Beconase **BECLOMETHASONE** glucocorticoid
Bemote **DICYCLOMINE** antispasmodic
Benadryl **DIPHENHYDRAMINE** antihistamine
BENAZAPRIL Lotensin antihypertensive
BENDROFLUMETHIAZIDE Naturetin diuretic
Benemid **PROBENECID** antigout
Benicar **OLMESARTAN** hypertension
Bentyl **DICYCLOMINE** antispasmodic
BENZONATATE Tessalon antitussive
BENZQUINAMIDE Emete-con antiemetic
BENZTHIAZIDE Exna diuretic
BENZTROPINE Cogentin anti-Parkinson's
BEPRIDIL Vascor calcium channel blocker
BETACLOMETHASONE Beclovent, Becloforte, Qvar,
    Vanceril asthma
BETAINE Cystadane homocysteine antagonist
BETAMETHASONE glucocorticoid

Betapace **SOTALOL** β-blocker
Betaseron **INTERFERON 1B** multiple sclerosis
BETAXOLOL Kerlone β-blocker
BETHANECHOL Urecholine urinary retention
BEVACIZUMAB Avastin oncology
Bevitamel **MELATONIN** sleep hormone
Bextra **VALDECOXIB** NSAID
Biaxin **CLARITHROMYCIN** anti-infective
BICALTAMIDE Casodex oncology
BiCNU **CARMUSTINE** oncology
BIPERIDEN Akineton anti-Parkinson's
BISACODYL Dulcolax laxative
BISOPROLOL Zebeta β-blocker, antihypertensive
BITOLTEROL Tornalate bronchodilator, asthma
BIVALIRUDIN Angiomax anticoagulant
Blenoxane **BLEOMYCIN** antibiotic, antineoplastic
BLEOMYCIN Blenoxane antibiotic, antineoplastic
Blocadren **TIMOLOL** β-blocker
Bontril **PHENDIMETRAZINE** appetite suppressant
BOSENTAN Tracleer pulmonary hypertension
Botox **BOTULINUM** paralytic
BOTULINUM Botox paralytic
Brethine **TERBUTALINE** bronchodilator
Bravelle **UROFOLLITROPIN** infertility
Brevibloc **ESMOLOL** β-blocker
Bromfed **BROMPHENIRAMINE** antihistamine
BROMOCRIPTINE Parlodel anti-Parkinson's
BROMPHENIRAMINE Bromfed antihistamine
BROMPHENIRAMINE & PSEUDOEPHEDRINE
    Ultrabrom antihistamine
Bronkosol **ISOETHARINE** bronchodilator
BUDESONIDE Rhinocart glucocorticoid
BUMETANIDE Bumex loop diuretic
Bumex **BUMETANIDE** loop diuretic
Buprenex **BUPRENORPHINE** narcotic
BUPRENORPHINE Buprenex narcotic

BUPROPION Zyban, Wellbutrin antidepressant
BuSpar **BUSPIRONE** antianxiety agent
BUSPIRONE BuSpar antianxiety agent
BUTABARBITAL Butisol Sodium sedative
BUTALBITAL & ASA Fiorinal tension H/A
BUTENAFINE Mentax antifungal
Butisol Sodium **BUTABARBITAL** sedative
BUTOCONAZOLE Femstat antifungal
BUTORPHANOL Stadol narcotic
Byclomine **DICYCLOMINE** antispasmodic

CABERGOLINE Dostinex anti-hyperprolactinemic
Caduet **AMIODIPINE/ATORVASTATIN** angina
Caelyx **DOXORUBICIN** breast cancer
Cafergot **ERGOTAMINE** migraine and vascular H/A
Calan **VERAPAMIL** calcium channel blocker
Calcibind **CELLULOSE SODIUM PHOSPHATE**
    prevents kidney stones
CALCIFEDIOL Calderol vitamin D supplement
CALCITONIN Miacalcin osteoporosis
CALCIRIOL Rocaltrol vitamin D supplement
Calderol **CALCIFEDIOL** vitamin D supplement
Camila **NORETHINDRONE** oral contraceptive
Camptosar **IRINOTECAN** colorectal cancer
Canasa **MESALAMINE** Crohn's disease
CANDESARTAN CILEXETIL Atacand hypertension
CAPECITABINE Xeloda oncology
Capoten **CAPTOPRIL** antihypertensive, ACE inhibitor
Capozide **HCTZ & CAPTOPRIL** antihypertensive
CAPTOPRIL Capoten antihypertensive, ACE inhibitor
Carac **FLUOROURACIL** oncology
Carafate **SUCRALFATE** antiulcer
CARBAMAZEPINE Atretiol, Carbatrol, Tegretol
    anticonvulsant
Carbatrol **CARBAMAZEPINE** anticonvulsant
CARBENICILLIN Geocillin antibiotic

CARBETAPENTANE Rynatuss cough
CARBIDOPA Lodosyn Parkinson's
CARBINOXAMINE Rondec antihistamine
Cardene **NICARDIPINE** antianginal, calcium channel blocker
Cardizem **DILTIAZEM** antianginal, calcium channel blocker
Cardura **DOXAZOSIN** antihypertensive
CARISOPRODOL Soma muscle relaxant
CARMUSTINE BiCNU, Gliadel Wafer oncology
CARTEOLOL Cartrol β-blocker
Cartia **DILTIAZEM** calcium channel blocker
Cartrol **CARTEOLOL** β-blocker
CARVEDILOL Coreg alpha and β-blocker
Casodex **BICALTAMIDE** oncology
Cataflam **DICLOFENAC** NSAID
Catapres **CLONIDINE** antihypertensive
Caverject **ALPROSTADIL** erectile dysfunction
Ceclor **CEFACLOR** antibiotic
Cedax **CEFTIBUTEN** antibiotic
CeeNU **LOMUSTINE** oncology
CEFACLOR Ceclor antibiotic
CEFADROXIL Duricef antibiotic
CEFAZOLIN Ancef, Kefzol antibiotic
CEFDINIR Omnicef antibiotic
CEFDITOREN Spectracef antibiotic
CEFIXIME Suprax antibiotic
Cefizox **CEFTIZOXIME** antibiotic
CEFMETAZOLE Zefazone antibiotic
CEFOTAXIME Claforan antibiotic
CEFOXITIN Mefoxin antibiotic
CEFPODOXIME PROXETIL Vantin antibiotic
CEFPROZIL Cefzil cephalosporin antibiotic
CEFTAZIDIME Taxidime antibiotic
CEFTIBUTEN Cedax antibiotic
Ceftin **CEFUROXIME** antibiotic

CEFTIZOXIME Cefizox antibiotic
CEFTRIAXONE Rocephin antibiotic
CEFUROXIME Ceftin antibiotic
Cefzil **CEFPROZIL** cephalosporin antibiotic
Celebrex **CELECOXIB** anti-inflammatory
CELECOXIB Celebrex anti-inflammatory
Celestone **BETAMETHASONE** steroid
Celexa **CITALOPRAM** depression
CellCept **MYCOPHENOLATE** immunosuppressant
CELLULOSE SODIUM PHOSPHATE Calcibind
      prevents kidney stones
Celontin **METHSUXIMIDE** anticonvulsant
Cenestin **ESTROGEN** hormone
Centrax **PRAZEPAM** sedative, benzodiazepine
CEPHALEXIN Keflex antibiotic
CEPHRADINE Velosef antibiotic
Cerebyx **FOSPHENYTOIN** status epilepticus
CERIVASTATIN Baycol elevated cholesterol
Cetamide **SULFACETAMIDE** antifungal
CETIRIZINE Zyrtec antihistamine
CETRORELIX Cetrotide hormone
Cetrotide **CETRORELIX** hormone
CETUXIMAB Erbitux oncology
Chantix **VARENICLINE** smoking cessation
Chlo-Amine **CHLORPHENIRAMINE** antihistamine
CHLORAL HYDRATE sedative
CHLORAMBUCIL Leukeran anti-inflammatory
CHLORAMPHENICOL Chlorofair antibiotic
CHLORDIAZEPOXIDE Librium benzodiazepine
CHLORDIAZEPOXIDE & AMITRIPTYLINE Limbitrol
      antianxiety agent, antidepressant
CHLORDIAZEPOXIDE & CLIDINIUM Librax
      benzodiazepine, anticholinergic
CHLORMEZANONE Trancopal antianxiety agent
Chlorofair **CHLORAMPHENICOL** antibiotic
CHLOROTHIAZIDE Diuril diuretic, antihypertensive

CHLOROTRIANISENE Tace estrogen
CHLORPHENESIN Maolate muscle relaxant
CHLORPHENIRAMINE Chlor-Trimeton, Aller-Chlor, Chlo-Amine antihistamine
CHLORPROMAZINE Thorazine antipsychotic
CHLORPROPAMIDE Diabinese hypoglycemic agent
CHLORTHALIDONE Hygroton diuretic
Chlor-Trimeton **CHLORPHENIRAMINE** antihistamine
CHLORZOXAZONE Paraflex sedative
Choledyl **THEOPHYLLINE** bronchodilator
CHOLESTRYRAMINE LoCholest antilipemic
CHOLINE MAGNESIUM TRISALICYLATE Trilisate non-narcotic analgesic
CHOLINE SALICYLATE Arthropan non-narcotic analgesic
CHORIONIC GONADOTROPIN Ovidrel ovulation stimulator
CICLOPIROX OLAMINE Loprox antifungal
CILOSTAZOL Pletal intermittent claudication
CIMETIDINE Tagamet antiulcer
Cinobac **CINOXACIN** antibiotic
CINOXACIN Cinobac, Pulvules antibiotic
Cipro **CIPROFLOXACIN** antibiotic
CIPROFLOXACIN Cipro antibiotic
CISAPRIDE Propulsid GI prokinetic agent
CISPLATIN Platinol oncology
CITALOPRAM Celexa depression
CLADRIBINE Leustatin antineoplastic
Claforan **CEFOTAXIME** antibiotic
CLARITHROMYCIN Biaxin anti-infective
Claritin **LORATADINE** antihistamine
CLEMASTINE Tavist antihistamine
Cleocin **CLINDAMYCIN** anti-infective
Climara **ESTRADIOL TRANSDERMAL** osteoporosis
CLINDAMYCIN Cleocin anti-infective
Clinoril **SULINDAC** NSAID

CLOBETASOL Cormax corticosteroid
CLOFAZIMINE Lamprene anti-infective
CLOFIBRATE Abitrate anti-hyperlipidemic
Clomid **CLOMIPHENE** hormone
CLOMIPHENE Clomid, Serophene hormone
CLOMIPRAMINE Anafranil tricyclic antidepressant
CLONAZEPAM Klonopin anticonvulsant
CLONIDINE Catapres antihypertensive
CLOPIDROGREL Plavix antiplatelet agent
CLORAZEPATE Tranxene antianxiety
CLOTRIMAZOLE Lotrimin, Mycelex antifungal
CLOXACILLIN Cloxapen antibiotic
Cloxapen **CLOXACILLIN** antibiotic
CLOZAPINE Clozaril antipsychotic
Clozaril **CLOZAPINE** antipsychotic
CODEINE narcotic analgesic, antitussive
Cogentin **BENZTROPINE** anti-Parkinson's
Cognex **TACRINE** Alzheimer's dementia
Colace **DOCUSATE** laxative
Colazal **BALSALAZIDE** anti-inflammatory
COLESEVELAM WelChol anti-lipemic
Colestid **COLESTIPOL** lipid-lowering agent
COLCHICINE antigout agent
COLESTIPOL Colestid lipid-lowering agent
COLISTIN Polymyxin E antibiotic
CombiPatch **ESTRADIOL** hormone
Combivent **ALBUTEROL & IPRATROPIUM**
   bronchodilators
Combivir **LAMIVUDINE & ZIDOVUDINE** antivirals
Compazine **PROCHLORPERAZINE** antiemetic
Comtan **ENTACAPONE** anti-Parkinson's
Concerta **METHYLPHENIDATE** stimulant ADHD
Condylox **PODOFILOX** genital warts
Copaxone **GLATIRAMER** multiple sclerosis
Cordarone **AMIODARONE** refractory VTach
Coreg **CARVEDILOL** alpha and β-blocker

Corgard **NADOLOL** antihypertensive, β-blocker
Corlopam **FENOLDOPAM MESYLATE** hypertension
Cormax **CLOBETASOL** corticosteroid
CORTISONE steroid
Cosmegen **DACTINOMYCIN** antineoplastic
Cosopt **DORZOLAMIDE & TIMOLOL** β-blocker
CO-TRIMOXAZOLE Bactrim antibiotic
Coumadin **WARFARIN** anticoagulant
Cozaar **LOSARTAN** hypertension
Crixivan **INDINAVIR** HIV
CROMOLYN Intal, Nasalcrom allergic rhinitis
Cuprimine **PENICILLAMINE** anti-inflammatory
CYCLOBENZAPRINE Flexeril skeletal muscle relaxant
CYCLOPHOSPHAMIDE Cytoxan anti-inflammatory
CYCLOSPORINE Sandimmune immunosuppressant
Cylert **PEMOLINE** CNS stimulant
Cymbalta **DULOXETINE** antidepressant
Cystadane **BETAINE** homocysteine antagonist
Cystospaz **HYOSCYAMINE** stomach disorders
Cytomel **LIOTHYRONINE** antihypothyroidism agent
Cytotec **MISOPROSTOL** antiulcer
Cytovene **GANCICLOVIR** antiviral
Cytoxan **CYCLOPHOSPHAMIDE** anti-inflammatory

D4T STAVUDINE Zerit antiviral
DACTINOMYCIN Cosmegen antineoplastic
Dalmane **FLURAZEPAM** sedative, benzodiazepine
DANAZOL Danocrine hormone
Danocrine **DANAZOL** hormone
Dantrium **DANTROLENE** skeletal muscle relaxant
DANTROLENE Dantrium skeletal muscle relaxant
Daranide **DICHLORPHENAMIDE** glaucoma
Daraprim **PYRIMETHAMINE** malaria
Darvon **PROPOXYPHENE** narcotic
DAUNORUBICIN Daunoxome oncology
Daunoxome **DAUNORUBICIN** oncology

Daypro **OXAPROZIN** NSAID
Dazamide **ACETAZOLAMIDE** diuretic, anticonvulsant
Decadron **DEXAMETHASONE** glucocorticoid,
    anti-inflammatory agent
Deca-Durabolin **NANDROLONE** anemia, oncology
Declomycin **DEMECLOCYCLINE** antibiotic
DELAVIRDINE Rescriptor antiviral
Deltasone **PREDNISONE** corticosteroid
Demadex **TORSEMIDE** diuretic
DEMECLOCYCLINE Declomycin antibiotic
Demerol **MEPERIDINE** narcotic analgesic
Demser **METYROSINE** antihypertensive
Denavir **PENCICLOVIR** antiviral
Depacon **DIVALPROEX** epilepsy
Depade **NALTREXONE** opioid antidote
Depakene **VALPROIC ACID** anticonvulsant
Depakote **DIVALPROEX SODIUM** anticonvulsant, H/A
Depen **PENICILLAMINE** anti-inflammatory
Depo-Medrol **METHYLPREDNISOLONE** steroid
Depo-Provera **MEDROXYPROGESTERONE** hormone
Deprenyl **SELEGILINE** MAO inhibitor
DES **DIETHYLSTILBESTROL** hormone
DESIPRAMINE Norpramin tricyclic antidepressant
DESONIDE Desowen steroid
Desowen **DESONIDE** steroid
Desyrel **TRAZODONE** antidepressant
Detrol **TOLTERODINE** overactive bladder
Dexadrine **DEXTROAMPHETAMINE** CNS stimulant
DEXAMETHASONE Decadron glucocorticoid,
    anti-inflammatory agent
DEXMETHYLPHENIDATE Focalin ADHD
DEXTROAMPHETAMINE Dexadrine CNS stimulant
Dextrostat **DEXTROAMPHETAMINE** ADHD
DHE 45 **DIHYDROERGOTAMINE** vascular H/A
DHPG **GANCICLOVIR** antiviral
Diabeta **GLYBURIDE** hypoglycemic agent

Diabinese **CHLORPROPAMIDE** hypoglycemic agent
Diamox **ACETAZOLAMIDE** diuretic, anticonvulsant
DIAZEPAM Valium benzodiazepine, sedative
DIAZOXIDE Hyperstat acute hypertension
Dibenzyline **PHENOXYBENZAMINE** antihypertensive
DICHLORLPHENAZONE Midrin H/A
DICHLORPHENAMIDE Daranide glaucoma
DICLOFENAC Cataflam, Voltaren NSAID
DICLOXACILLIN Dynapen antibiotic
DICYCLOMINE Bemote, Bentyl, Byclomine
    antispasmodic
DIDANOSINE Videx antiviral
Didronel **ETIDRONATE** osteoporosis
DIETHYLPROPION Tenuate obesity
DIETHYLSTILBESTROL DES hormone
DIFENOXIN Motofen antidiarrheal
Differin **ADAPALENE** acne
DIFLORASONE Psorcon steroid
Diflucan **FLUCONAZOLE** antifungal
DIFLUNISAL Dolobid NSAID, non-narcotic analgesic
Digibind **DIGOXIN IMMUNE FAB** antidote for digoxin
DIGOXIN Lanoxin inotrope, antiarrhythmic
DIGOXIN IMMUNE FAB Digibind antidote for digoxin
DIHYDROCODEINE Synalgos narcotic
DIHYDROERGOTAMINE DHE 45 vascular H/A
Dilatrate **ISOSORBIDE** angina, nitrate
DILTIAZEM Cardizem, Cartia antianginal, calcium
    channel blocker
Dilantin **PHENYTOIN** anticonvulsant
Dilaudid **HYDROMORPHINE** narcotic analgesic
DIMENHYDRINATE Dramamine antiemetic
Diovan **VALSARTAN** hypertension
Dipentum **OLSALAZINE** GI anti-inflammatory
DIPHENHYDRAMINE Benadryl antihistamine
DIPHENOXYLATE Lomotil antidiarrheal
DIPYRIDAMOLE Persantin antiplatelet agent

DIRITHROMYCIN Dynabac antibiotic
DISOPYRAMIDE Norpace antiarrhythmic
DISULFIRAM Antabuse alcohol abuse deterrent
Ditropan **OXYBUTYNIN CHLORIDE** overactive bladder
Diucardin **HYDROFLUMETHIAZIDE** diuretic
Diuril **CHLOROTHIAZIDE** diuretic, antihypertensive
DIVALPROEX Depakote, Depacon anticonvulsant
DNASE Pulmozyme cystic fibrosis
DOBUTAMINE Dobutrex inotrope
Dobutrex **DOBUTAMINE** inotrope
DOCUSATE Colace laxative
DOFETILIDE Tikosyn antiarrhythmic
DOLASETRON Anzemet antiemetic
Dolobid **DIFLUNISAL** NSAID, non-narcotic analgesic
Dolophine **METHADONE** narcotic
DONEPEZIL Aricept Alzheimer's disease
Donnamar **HYOSCYAMINE** stomach disorders
Donnatal **PHENOBARBITAL & ATROPINE**
    antidiarrheal
DOPAMINE Intropin vasopressor, inotrope
Dopar **LEVODOPA** anti-Parkinson's
Doral **QUAZEPAM** benzodiazepine
DORNASE ALFA Pulmozyme mucolytic
DORZOLAMIDE Trusopt glaucoma
Dostinex **CABERGOLINE** anti-hyperprolactinemic
DOXAZOSIN Cardura antihypertensive
DOXEPIN Sinaquan, Adapin tricyclic antidepressant
DOXERCALCIFEROL Hectorol reduces parathyroid
    hormone levels
DOXORUBICIN Adriamycin, Caelyx oncology
Doxy **DOXYCYCLINE** antibiotic
DOXYCYCLINE Vibramycin, Doxy antibiotic
DOXYLAMINE Unisom sedative
Dramamine **DIMENHYDRINATE** antiemetic
DRONABINOL Marinol nausea
DROPERIDOL Inapsine antiemetic, tranquilizer

DROTRECOGIN ALFA Xigris sepsis
Dulcolax **BISACODYL** laxative
DULOXETINE Cymbalta antidepressant
Duragen **ESTRADIOL** hormone
Duragesic **FENTANYL TRANSDERMAL** narcotic
    analgesic
Duricef **CEFADROXIL** antibiotic
Dycill **DICLOXICILLIN** antibiotic
Dymelor **ACETOHEXAMIDE** diabetes
Dynabac **DIRITHROMYCIN** antibiotic
Dynacin **MINOCYCLINE** antibiotic
DynaCirc **ISRADIPINE** antihypertensive
Dynapen **DICLOXACILLIN** antibiotic
DYPHYLLINE Asminyl bronchodilator
Dyrenium **TRIAMTERENE** diuretic

E-mycin **ERYTHROMYCIN** antibiotic
ECONAZOLE Spectazole antifungal
Edecrin **ETHACRYNIC ACID** hypertension, CHF
Edex **ALPROSTADIL** anti-impotence agent
EDROPHONIUM Tensilon cholinergic-
    anti-cholinesterase
ED-SPAZ **HYOSCYAMINE** stomach disorders
EFAVIRENZ Sustiva antiviral
Effexor **VENLAFAXINE** antidepressant
EFLORNITHINE Vaniqa hair growth inhibitor
Efudex **FLUOROURACIL** oncology
E-Lor **PROPOXYPHENE & ACETAMINOPHEN** pain
    control
Eldepryl **SELEGILINE** anti-Parkinson's
ELETRIPTAN Relpax migraine
Eligard **LEUPROLIDE** oncology
Elitek **RASBURICASE** uric acid reducer
Ellence **EPIRUBICIN** breast cancer
Elmiron **PENTOSAN POLYSULFATE**
    anti-inflammatory

Eloxatin **OXALIPLATIN** oncology
Elspar **ASPARAGINASE** oncology
Eltroxin **LEVOTHYROXINE** thyroid
Emcyt **ESTRAMUSTINE** prostate cancer
Emete-con **BENZQUINAMIDE** antiemetic
Eminase **ANISTREPLASE** thrombolytic
ENALAPRIL Vasotec antihypertensive
Enbrel **ETANERCEPT** anti-inflammatory
Enduron **METHYCLOTHIAZIDE** diuretic
ENOXACIN Penetrex anti-infective
ENOXAPRARIN Lovenox antithrombotic
ENTACAPONE Comtan Parkinson's
Entocort EC **BUDESONIDE** Crohn's
EPIRUBICIN Ellence breast cancer
Epitol **CARBAMAZEPINE** antiepileptic
Epivir **LAMIVUDINE** anti-infective
EPLERENONE Inspra hypertension
EPOPROSTENOL Flolan pulmonary hypertension
EPROSARTAN Teveten hypertension
EPTIFIBATIDE Integrilin anticoagulant
Equanil **MEPROBAMATE** sedative
Erbitux **CETUXIMAB** oncology
Ercaf **ERGOTAMINE** migraine
Ergamisol **LEVAMISOLE** oncology
ERGOLOID Gerimal stimulates brain cells
Ergomar **ERGOTAMINE** migraine
Ergostat **ERGOTAMINE** migraine
ERGOTAMINE Cafergot, Ergostat, Wigraine migraine
Erythrocin **ERYTHROMYCIN** antibiotic
ERYTHROMYCIN E-mycin antibiotic
Eryzole **ERYTHROMYCIN** antibiotic
ESCITALOPRAM Lexapro antidepressant
Esidrix **HYDROCHLOROTHIAZIDE** diuretic
ESMOLOL Brevibloc β-blocker
ESOMEPRAZOLE Nexium gastric reflux
ESTAZOLAM ProSom sedative, benzodiazepine

Estrace **ESTRADIOL** hormone
ESTRADIOL Alora, Estrace, Activella, Vagifem, Vivelle hormone
ESTRADIOL TRANSDERMAL Climara osteoporosis
ESTRAMUSTINE Emcyt prostate cancer
ESTROPIPATE Ogen hormone
ETANERCEPT Enbrel anti-inflammatory
ETHACRYNIC ACID Edecrin hypertension, CHF
ETHCHLORVYNOL Placidyl sedative
Ethmozine **MORICIZINE** antiarrhythmic
ETHOSUXIMIDE Zarontin anticonvulsant
ETHOTOIN Peganone anticonvulsant
Ethyol **AMIFOSTINE** oncology
ETIDRONATE Didronel osteoporosis
ETODOLAC Lodine NSAID
Etrafon **PERPHENAZINE & AMITRIPTYLINE** tricyclic antidepressant
Eulexin **FLUTAMIDE** oncology
E-Vista **RALOXIFENE** osteoporosis
Exelon **RIVASTIGMINE** Alzheimer's
EXEMESTANE Aromasin breast cancer
Exna **BENZTHIAZIDE** diuretic
EZETIMIBE Zetia anti-lipemic
Ezide **HYDROCHLOROTHIAZIDE** diuretic

FAMCICLOVIR Famvir antiviral
FAMOTIDINE Pepcid antiulcer
Famvir **FAMCICLOVIR** antiviral
Fareston **TOREMIFENE** oncology
Faslodex **FULVESTRANT** breast cancer
Fastin **PHENTERMINE** anorexiant
FELBAMATE Felbatol anticonvulsant
Felbatol **FELBAMATE** anticonvulsant
Feldene **PIROXICAM** NSAID
FELODIPINE Plendil calcium channel blocker, antihypertensive

Femara **LETROZOLE** breast cancer
FemHrt **ESTRADIOL & NORETHINDRONE** osteoporosis
Femstat **BUTOCONAZOLE** antifungal
FENOFIBRATE Lipidil lipid-lowering agent
FENOLDOPAM MESYLATE Corlopam hypertensive
    crisis
FENOPROFEN Nalfon NSAID
FENTANYL Sublimaze narcotic analgesic
FENTANYL TRANSDERMAL Duragesic narcotic
Fertinex **UROFOLLITIN** induces ovulation
FEXOFENADINE Allegra antihistamine
FILGRASTIM Neupogen anti-inflammatory
FINASTERIDE Proscar enzyme inhibitor
Fioricet **BUTALBITAL & ACETAMINOPHEN** migraine
Fiorinal **BUTALBITAL & ASA** tension H/A
FK-506 TACROLIMUS Fujimycin, Prograf
    immunosuppressant
Flagyl **METRONIDAZOLE** antibiotic
FLAVOXATE Urispas bladder antispasmodic
FLECAINIDE Tambocor antiarrhythmic
Flexeril **CYCLOBENZAPRINE** skeletal muscle relaxant
Flolan **EPOPROSTENOL** pulmonary hypertension
Flomax **TAMSULOSIN** prostatic hyperplasia
Flonase **FLUTICASONE PROPIONATE** anti-allergic
Flovent **FLUTICASONE** asthma: steroid inhaler
Floxin **OFLOXACIN** antibiotic
FLUCONAZOLE Diflucan antifungal
FLUCYTOSINE Ancobon antifungal
Fludara **FLUDARABINE** oncology
FLUDARABINE Fludara oncology
Flumadine **RIMANTADINE** antiviral
FLUMAZENIL Romazicon benzodiazepine antagonist
FLUNISOLIDE Aerobid steroid
FLUOCINONIDE Lidex steroid
FLUOROURACIL Adrucil, Carac, Efudex oncology
Fluoroplex **FLUOROURACIL** oncology

FLUOXETINE Prozac antidepressant
FLUOXYMESTERONE Android-F oncology
FLUPHENAZINE Prolixin antipsychotic, phenothiazine
FLURAZEPAM Dalmane sedative, benzodiazepine
FLURBIPROFEN Ansaid NSAID
FLUTICASONE/SALMETEROL Advair DisKus steroid
FLUTICASONE PROPIONATE Flonase anti-allergic
FLUTAMIDE Eulexin oncology
FLUVASTATIN Lescol cholesterol-lowering agent
FLUVOXAMINE Luvox antidepressant
Focalin **DEXMETHYLPHENIDATE** ADHD
Folex **METHOTREXATE** psoriasis, arthritis
Follistim **FOLLITROPIN** fertility therapy
FOLLITROPIN Follistim fertility therapy
Foradil **FORMOTEROL** asthma
FORMOTEROL Foradil asthma
Forteo **TERIPARATIDE** osteoporosis
Fortovase **SAQUINAVIR** antiviral
Fosamax **ALENDRONATE** osteoporosis
FOSAMPRENAVIR Lexiva antiretroviral
FOSCARNET Foscavir antiviral AIDS
Foscavir **FOSCARNET** antiviral AIDS
FOSFOMYCIN Monurol antibiotic UTI
FOSINOPRIL Monopril antihypertensive
FOSPHENYTOIN Cerebyx status epilepticus
Frova **FROVATRIPTAN** migraine
FROVATRIPTAN Frova migraine
Fujimycin **FK-506 TACROLIMUS** immunosuppressant
FULVESTRANT Faslodex breast cancer
Fulvicin **GRISEOFULVIN** antifungal
Fumide **FUROSEMIDE** diuretic
FUROSEMIDE Lasix, Fumide diuretic

GABAPENTIN Neurontin anticonvulsant
Gabitril **TIAGABINE** epilepsy
GALANTAMINE Reminyl Alzheimer's

GANCICLOVIR Cytovene, Vitrasert antiviral
Gantrisin **SULFISOXAZOLE** antibiotic
Garamycin **GENTAMICIN** antibiotic
Gastrocrom **CROMOLYN** asthma
Gastroseda **HYOSCYAMINE** stomach disorders
GATIFLOXACIN Tequin antibiotic
GELSEMIUM neuralgia, cold sx
GEMCITABINE Gemzar pancreatic cancer
GEMFIBROZIL Lopid lipid-lowering agent
GAMMA-HYDROXYBUTRATE GHB sedative
Gemzar **GEMCITABINE** pancreatic cancer
Gengraf **CYCLOSPORINE** immunosuppressant
GENTAMICIN Garamycin antibiotic
Geocillin **CARBENICILLIN** antibiotic
Geodon **ZIPRASIDONE** schizophrenia
Gerimal **ERGOLOID** stimulates brain cells
GHB GAMMA-HYDROXYBUTRATE sedative
GLATIRAMER Copaxone multiple sclerosis
Gleevec **IMATINIB** oncology
Gliadel Wafer **CARMUSTINE** oncology
GLIMEPIRIDE Amaryl diabetes
GLIPIZIDE Glucotrol hypoglycemic agent
GLUCAGON hormone, antidiabetic agent
Glucophage **METFORMIN** type II diabetes
Glucotrol **GLIPIZIDE** hypoglycemic agent
GLYBURIDE Diabeta, Micronase hypoglycemic agent
Glynase **GLYBURIDE** hypoglycemic agent
Glyset **MIGLITOL** diabetes
Golytely **POLYETHYLENE GLYCOL** constipation
GOSERELIN ACETATE Zoladex oncology
GRANISETRON Kytril antiemetic
Gravol **DIMENHYDRINATE** antihistamine
GREPAFLOXACIN Raxar anti-infective
Grisactin **GRISEOFULVIN** antibiotic
GRISEOFULVIN Fulvicin, Grisactin antibiotic
GUAIFENESIN cough preparation

GUANABENZ Wytensin antihypertensive
GUANADREL Hylorel antihypertensive
GUANETHIDINE Ismelin antihypertensive
GUANFACINE Tenex antihypertensive

HALAZEPAM Paxipam sedative, benzodiazepine
Halcion **TRIAZOLAM** sedative, benzodiazepine
Haldol **HALOPERIDOL** antipsychotic
Halfan **HALOFANTRINE** antimalarial
HALOBETASOL Ultravate steroid
HALOFANTRINE Halfan antimalarial
HALOPERIDOL Haldol antipsychotic
HALOPROGIN Halotex antifungal
Halotex **HALOPROGIN** antifungal
HCTZ diuretic
Hectorol **DOXERCALCIFEROL** reduces parathyroid
   hormone levels
HEPARIN anticoagulant
Herceptin **TRASTUZUMAB** oncology
Hexadrol **DEXAMETHASONE** steroid
Hexalen **ALTRERAMINE** oncology
Hiprex **METHENAMINE** antibiotic
Hivid **ZALCITABINE** anti-infective
HMG **MENOTROPINS** hormone
Humalog **INSULIN LISPRO** diabetes mellitus
Humatrope **SOMATROPIN** growth hormone
Humira **ADALIMUMAB** rheumatoid arthritis
Humulin **INSULIN** diabetes
Hycamtin **TOPOTECAN** oncology
Hydergine **ERGOLOID** stimulates brain cells
HYDRALAZINE Apresoline antihypertensive
Hydrea **HYDROXYUREA** sickle-cell anemia
HYDROCHLOROTHIAZIDE Aquazide, Hydrodiuril
   diuretic
Hydrocil **PSYLLIUM** constipation

HYDROCODONE Anexsia, Lortab, Vicodin narcotic analgesic

HYDROCODONE & IBUPROFEN Vicoprofen narcotic analgesic, NSAID

HYDROCORTISONE Solu-Cortef glucocorticoid, short-acting

Hydrodiuril **HYDROCHLOROTHIAZIDE** diuretic

HYDROFLUMETHIAZIDE Diucardin, Saluron diuretic

HYDROMORPHINE Dilaudid narcotic analgesic

HYDROXYUREA Hydrea sickle-cell anemia

HYDROXYZINE Anxanil, Atarax, Vistaril, Vistaject sedative

Hygroton **CHLORTHALIDONE** diuretic

Hylorel **GUANADREL** antihypertensive

HYOSCYAMINE Anaspaz, A-Spas, Cystopaz, Donnamar, ED-SPAZ, Gastroseda, Levbid, Levsin stomach disorders

Hyperstat **DIAZOXIDE** acute hypertension

Hytrin **TERAZOSIN** antihypertensive

Hyzaar **LOSARTAN & HCTZ** hypertension

Hyzine-50 **HYDROXYZINE** sedative

IBUPROFEN Advil, Motrin, Nuprin NSAID

Idamycin **IDARUBICIN** antineoplastic

IDARUBICIN Idamycin antineoplastic

IMATINIB Gleevec oncology

Imdur **ISOSORBIDE MONOITRATE** vasodilator

IMIPENEM Primaxin antibiotic

IMIPRAMINE Tofranil tricyclic antidepressant

IMIQUIMOD Aldara anti-inflammatory

Imitrex **SUMATRIPTAN** migraine

Imodium **LOPERAMIDE** antidiarrheal

Imuran **AZATHIOPRINE** immunosuppressant

Inapsine **DROPERIDOL** antiemetic, tranquilizer

INDAPAMIDE Lozol diuretic

Inderal **PROPRANOLOL** antihypertensive, β-blocker
Inderide **PROPRANOLOL** antihypertensive, β-blocker
INDINAVIR Crixivan HIV
Indocin **INDOMETHACIN** NSAID
INDOMETHACIN Indocin NSAID
INFLIXIMAB Remicade Crohn's disease
Inocor **AMRINONE** inotropic agent
Inspra **EPLERENONE** hypertension
INSULIN LISPRO Humalog diabetes mellitus
Intal **CROMOLYN SODIUM** asthma, allergic rhinitis
Integrilin **EPTIFIBATIDE** anticoagulant
INTERFERON antineoplastic
INTERFERON 1B Betaseron multiple sclerosis
Intropin **DOPAMINE** vasopressor, inotrope
Invirase **SAQUINAVIR** anti-infective
Ionamin **PHENTERMINE** appetite suppressant
IPRATROPIUM Atrovent bronchodilator
IRBESARTAN Avapro hypertension
IRINOTECAN Camtosar oncology
Ismelin **GUANETHIDINE** antihypertensive
Ismo **ISOSORBIDE MONONITRATE** vasodilator
ISOCARBOXAZID Marplan antidepressant
ISOETHARINE Bronkosol bronchodilator
Isoptin **VERAPAMIL** calcium channel blocker
ISOPROTERENOL Isuprel inotrope, bronchodilator
Isordil **ISOSORBIDE DINITRATE** vasodilator
ISOSORBIDE DINITRATE Isordil vasodilator
ISOSORBIDE MONONITRATE Ismo vasodilator
ISOTRETINOIN Accutane antiacne agent
ISRADIPINE DynaCirc antihypertensive
Isuprel **ISOPROTERENOL** inotrope, bronchodilator
ITRACONAZOLE Sporanox anti-infective
IVERMECTIN Stromectol anti-parasite

Jenest-28 **NORETHINDRONE & ESTRADIOL** hormone

Kadian **MORPHINE** narcotic
Kaletra **LOPINAVIR & RITONAVIR** antiviral
Kaopectate **BISMUTH SUBSALICYLATE** antidiarrheal
K-Dur **POTASSIUM** electrolyte
Keflex **CEPHALEXIN** antibiotic
Keftab **CEPHALEXIN** antibiotic
Kefzol **CEFAZOLIN** antibiotic
Kemadrin **PROCYCLIDINE** Parkinson's
Kenalog **TRIAMCINOLONE** steroid
Keppra **LEVETIRACETAM** epilepsy
Kerlone **BETAXOLOL** β-blocker
Ketalar **KETAMINE** general anesthetic
KETAMINE Ketalar general anesthetic
Ketek **TELITHROMYCIN** antibiotic
KETOCONAZOLE Nizoral antifungal
KETOPROFEN Actron, Orudis NSAID
KETOROLAC Acular Ophthalmic NSAID
KETOROLAC Toradol NSAID, non-narcotic analgesic
KETOTIFEN Zaditor antihistamine
Kineret **ANAKINRA** anti-rheumatic
Klonopin **CLONAZEPAM** anticonvulsant
K-Lor **POTASSIUM** electrolyte
Kytril **GRANISETRON** antiemetic

L-Dopa **LEVODOPA** anti-Parkinson's
LABETALOL Normodyne, Trandate β-blocker
Lamictal **LAMOTRIGINE** antiepileptic
Lamisil **TERBINAFINE** anti-infective
LAMIVUDINE 3TC Epivir anti-infective
LAMOTRIGINE Lamictal antiepileptic
Lamprene **CLOFAZIMINE** anti-infective
Lanoxicaps **DIGOXIN** inotrope, antiarrhythmic
Lanoxin **DIGOXIN** inotrope, antiarrhythmic
LANSOPRAZOLE Prevacid gastrointestinal
Lanvis **THIOGUANINE** oncology
Largactil **PHENOTHIAZINE** antipsychotic

Larodopa **LEVODOPA** Parkinson's
Lasix **FUROSEMIDE** diuretic
LATANOPROST Xalaton glaucoma
LEFLUNOMIDE Arava anti-inflammatory
Lescol **FLUVASTATIN** cholesterol-lowering agent
LETROZOLE Femara breast cancer
Leukeran **CHLORAMBUCIL** anti-inflammatory
LEUPROLIDE Lupron endometriosis, prostate cancer
Leustatin **CLADRIBINE** antineoplastic
LEVALBUTEROL Xopenex asthma
LEVAMISOLE Ergamisol oncology
Levaquin **LEVOFLOXACIN** anti-infective
Levatol **PENBUTOLOL** antihypertensive, β-blocker
Levbid **HYOSCYAMINE** bladder antispasmodic
LEVETIRACETAM Keppra epilepsy
Levitra **VARDENAFIL** erectile dysfunction
LEVODOPA L-Dopa, Dopar anti-Parkinson's
Levo-Dromoran **LEVORPHANOL** narcotic
LEVOFLOXACIN Levaquin anti-infective
Levophed **NOREPINEPHRINE** hypotension
LEVORPHANOL Levo-Dromoran narcotic
Levo-T **LEVOTHYROXINE** thyroid
Levothyroid **LEVOTHYROXINE** thyroid
LEVOTHYROXINE Eltroxin, Levothroid thyroid
Levoxyl **LEVOTHYROXINE** thyroid
Levsin **HYOSCYAMINE** stomach disorders
Levsinex **HYOSCYAMINE** sedative
Lexapro **ESCITALOPRAM** antidepressant
Lexiva **FOSAMPRENAVIR** antiretroviral
Lexxel **ENALAPRIL** ACE inhibitor
Librax **CHLORDIAZEPOXIDE & CLIDINIUM**
    benzodiazepine, anticholinergic
Librium **CHLORDIAZEPOXIDE** benzodiazepine
Lidex **FLUOCINONIDE** steroid
Limbitrol **CHLORDIAZEPOXIDE & AMITRIPTYLINE**
    antianxiety agent, antidepressant

Lincocin **LINCOMYCIN** antibiotic
LINCOMYCIN Lincocin antibiotic
LINEZOLID Zyvox antibacterial
LIOTHYRONINE Cytomel antihypothyroidism agent
LIOTRIX Thyrolar thyroid
Lioresal **BACLOFEN** skeletal muscle relaxant
Lipidil **FENOFIBRATE** lipid-lowering agent
Lipitor **ATORVASTATIN** elevated total cholesterol
LISINOPRIL Zestril ACE inhibitor
Lithostat **ACETOHYDROXAMIC ACID** UTI
LoCholest **CHOLESTRYRAMINE** antilipemic
Lodine **ETODOLAC** NSAID
Lodosyn **CARBIDOPA** Parkinson's
LOMEFLOXACIN Maxaquin antibiotic
LOMUSTINE CeeNU oncology
Lomotil **DIPHENOXYLATE & ATROPINE** antidiarrheal
LOPERAMIDE Imodium antidiarrheal
Lopid **GEMFIBROZIL** lipid-lowering agent
Lopressor **METOPROLOL** antihypertensive, β-blocker
Loprox **CICLOPIROX OLAMINE** antifungal
Lopurin **ALLOPURINOL** antigout
Lorabid **LORACARBEF** cephalosporin antibiotic
LORACARBEF Lorabid cephalosporin antibiotic
LORATADINE Claritin antihistamine
LORAZEPAM Ativan sedative, benzodiazepine
Lortab **ACETAMINOPHEN & HYDROCODONE**
    analgesic
LOSARTAN Cozaar, Hyzaar hypertension
Losec **OMEPRAZOLE** peptic ulcer disease
Lotensin **BENAZEPRIL** antihypertensive
Lotrel **AMLODIPINE & BENAZEPRIL** antihypertensive
Lotrimin **CLOTRIMAZOLE** antifungal
Lotrisone **CLOTRIMAZOLE** antifungal
Lotronex **ALOSETRON** Crohn's disease
LOVASTATIN Mevacor lipid-lowering agent
Lovenox **ENOXAPRARIN** antithrombotic

LOXAPINE Loxitane antipsychotic
Loxitane **LOXAPINE** antipsychotic
Lozol **INDAPAMIDE** diuretic
Ludiomil **MAPROTILINE** tricyclic antidepressant
Lupron **LEUPROLIDE** endometriosis, prostate cancer
Luvox **FLUVOXAMINE** antidepressant

Macrobid **NITROFURANTOIN** antibiotic
Macrodantin **NITROFURANTOIN** antibiotic
MALATHION Ovide lice
Mandelamine **METHENAMINE** UTI
Manerix **MOCLOBEMIDE** depression
Maolate **CHLORPHENESIN** muscle relaxant
MAPROTILINE Ludiomil tricyclic antidepressant
Marcillin **AMPICILLIN** antibiotic
Margesic **BUTALBITAL & ASA** analgesic
Marinol **DRONABINOL** nausea
Marplan **ISOCARBOXAZID** antidepressant
Matulane **PROCARBAZINE** oncology
Mavik **TRANDOLAPRIL** hypertension
Maxair **PIRBUTEROL** bronchodilator
Maxalt **RIZATRIPTAN** migraine
Maxaquin **LOMEFLOXACIN** antibiotic
Maxidone **HYDROCODONE** narcotic
Maxzide **TRIAMTERENE & HCTZ** diuretic
Mazanor **MAZINDOL** obesity
MAZINDOL Mazanor, Sanorex obesity
Mebaral **MEPHOBARBITAL** barbiturate, sedative
MECHLORETHAMINE Mustargen Hodgkin's
Meclan **MECLOCYCLINE** antibiotic
MECLIZINE Antivert antiemetic, vertigo
MECLOCYCLINE Meclan antibiotic
MECLOFENAMATE Meclomen NSAID
Meclomen **MECLOFENAMATE** NSAID
Medigesic **BUTALBITAL & ASA** analgesic
Medihaler **ERGOTAMINE** migraine

Medipren **IBUPROFEN** NSAID
Medrol **METHYLPREDNISOLONE** glucocorticoid
MEDROXYPROGESTERONE Depo-Provera hormone
MEFENAMIC ACID Ponstel NSAID
Mefoxin **CEFOXITIN** antibiotic
Megace **MEGESTROL** oncology
MEGESTROL Megace oncology
MELATONIN Bevtamel sleep hormone
Melfiat **PHENDIMETRAZINE** appetite suppressant
Mellaril **THIORIDAZINE** antipsychotic
MELOXICAM Mobic NSAID
MELPHALAN Alkeran anticancer agent
MEMANTINE Namenda Alzheimer's
Menest **ESTROGEN** hormone
MENOTROPINS HMG, Pergonal hormone
Mentax **BUTENAFINE** antifungal
MEPERIDINE Demerol narcotic analgesic
MEPHENYTOIN Mesantoin anticonvulsant
MEPHOBARBITAL Mebaral barbiturate, sedative
MEPROBAMATE Equanil sedative, antianxiety
Mepron **ATOVAQUONE** antibiotic
Meprospan **MEPROBAMATE** sedative, antianxiety
Meridia **SIBUTRAMINE** obesity
Meronem **MEROPENEM** antibiotic
MEROPENEM Meronem antibiotic
MESALAMINE Asacol, Canasa, Rowasa, Pentasa,
    Mesasal, Salofalk Crohn's disease
Mesantoin **MEPHENYTOIN** anticonvulsant
Mesasal **MESALAMINE** Crohn's disease
MESORIDAZINE Serentil antipsychotic
Mestinon **PYRIDOSTIGMINE** myasthenia gravis
Metadate **METHYLPHENIDATE** ADHD
Metaglip **GLIPIZIDE & METFORMIN** diabetes
Metahydrin **TRICHLORMETHIAZIDE** diuretic
METAPROTERENOL Alupent bronchodilator
METARAMINOL Aramine vasopressor

Metastron **STRONTIUM-89 CHLORIDE** analgesic
METAXALONE Skelaxin muscle relaxant
METFORMIN Apo-Metformin, Glucophage diabetes
METHADONE Dolophine, Methadose narcotic
Methadose **METHADONE** narcotic
METHAZOLAMIDE Neptazane antiglaucoma
METHENAMINE Hiprex antibiotic
METHICILLIN Staphcillin antibiotic
METHIMAZOLE Tapazole antithyroid agent
METHOCARBAMOL Robaxin skeletal muscle relaxant
METHOTREXATE Rheumatrex, Abitrexate
    anti-inflammatory
METHSUXIMIDE Celontin anticonvulsant
METHYCLOTHIAZIDE Enduron diuretic
METHYLDOPA Aldomet antihypertensive
METHYLPHENIDATE Concerta, Ritalin ADHD
METHYLPREDNISOLONE Depo-Medrol
    glucocorticoid
METHYLPREDNISOLONE SODIUM SUCCINATE
    Solu-Medrol glucocorticoid, intermediate-acting
METHYSERGIDE Sansert vascular headache
METOCLOPRAMIDE Reglan antiemetic
METOLAZONE Zaroxolyn diuretic, antihypertensive
METOPROLOL Lopressor antihypertensive, β-blocker
METRONIDAZOLE Flagyl antibiotic
METYROSINE Demser antihypertensive
Mevacor **LOVASTATIN** lipid-lowering agent
Mexate **METHOTREXATE** oncology
MEXILETINE Mexitil antiarrhythmic
Mexitil **MEXILETINE** antiarrhythmic
Mezlin **MEZLOCILLIN** antibiotic
MEZLOCILLIN Mezlin antibiotic
Miacalcin **CALCITONIN** osteoporosis
Micardis **TELMISARTAN** hypertension
Micatin **MICONAZOLE** antifungal
MICONAZOLE Monistat antifungal

Micronase **GLYBURIDE** blood glucose–lowering agent

Microzide **HCTZ** antihypertensive

MIDAMOR Amiloride diuretic

MIDAZOLAM Versed sedative, benzodiazepine

MIDODRINE ProAmatine orthostatic hypotension

Midrin **DICHLORLPHENAZONE** H/A

MIGLITOL Glyset diabetes

MILRINONE Primacor inotropic/vasodilator agent

Miltown **MEPROBAMATE** antianxiety agent

Minipress **PRAZOSIN** antihypertensive

Minizide **PRAZOSIN & POLYTHIAZIDE** hypertension

Minocin **MINOCYCLINE** antibiotic

MINOCYCLINE Minocin, Vectrin antibiotic

MINOXIDIL Rogaine hair-growing agent

Mintezol **THIABENDAZOLE** antiparasitic

Mirapex **PRAMIPEXOLE** Parkinson's disease

MIRTAZAPINE Remeron depression

MISOPROSTOL Cytotec antiulcer

Mithracin **PLICAMYCIN** antineoplastic

Mithramycin **PLICAMYCIN** antineoplastic

MITOXANTRONE Novantrone prostate cancer

Moban **MOLINDONE** antipsychotic

Mobic **MELOXICAM** NSAID

MOCLOBEMIDE Manerix depression

MODAFINIL Provigil narcolepsy

MOEXIPRIL Uniretic Univasc antihypertensive

MOLINDONE Moban antipsychotic

MOMETASONE Nasonex steroid

Monistat **MICONAZOLE** antifungal

Monodox **DOXYCYCLINE** antibiotic

Mono-Gesic **SALSALATE** NSAID, antipyretic

Monoket **ISOSORBIDE** antianginal

Monopril **FOSINOPRIL** antihypertensive

MONTELUKAST Singulair antiallergic

Monurol **FOSFOMYCIN** antibiotic

MORICIZINE Ethmozine antiarrhythmic

Motofen **DIFENOXIN & ATROPINE** antidiarrheal

Motrin **IBUPROFEN** NSAID

MOXIFLOXACIN Avelox antibiotic

Mucomyst **ACETYLCYSTEINE** antidote for acetaminophen overdose

MUPIROCIN Bactroban antibiotic

Muse **ALPROSTADIL** male impotence

Mustargen **MECHLORETHAMINE** Hodgkin's

Mycelex **CLOTRIMAZOLE** antifungal

Myciguent **NEOMYCIN** antibiotic

MYCOPHENOLATE CellCept immunosuppressant

Mycostatin **NYSTATIN** antifungal

Mysoline **PRIMIDONE** anticonvulsant

Mytelase **AMBENONIUM** myasthenia gravis

NABUMETONE Relafen NSAID

NADOLOL Corgard β-blocker

NAFARELIN Synarel hormone

Nafcil **NAFCILLIN** antibiotic

NAFCILLIN Nafcil antibiotic

NAFTIFINE Naftin antibiotic

Naftin **NAFTIFINE** antibiotic

NALBUPHINE Nubain narcotic

Nalfon **FENOPROFEN** NSAID

NALIDIXIC ACID NegGram antibiotic

NALMEFENE Revex narcotic antagonist

NALOXONE Narcan narcotic antagonist

NALTREXONE Depade opioid antidote

Namenda **MEMANTINE** Alzheimer's

NANDROLONE Deca-Durabolin anemia, oncology

Naprelan **NAPROXEN** NSAID

Naprosyn **NAPROXEN** NSAID

NAPROXEN Aleve, Naprosyn, Anaprox NSAID

NARATRIPTAN Amerge cluster headache in adults

Narcan **NALOXONE** narcotic antagonist

Nardil **PHENELZINE SULFATE** antidepressant
Nasalcrom **CROMOLYN SODIUM** asthma, allergic rhinitis
Nasarel **FLUNISOLIDE** steroid
Nasonex **MOMETASONE** steroid
Naturetin **BENDROFLUMETHIAZIDE** diuretic
Navane **THIOTHIXENE** antipsychotic
Navelbine **VINORELBINE** antineoplastic
NEDOCROMIL Tilade mast cell stabilizer
NEFAZODONE Serzone antidepressant
NegGram **NALIDIXIC ACID** antibiotic
NELFINAVIR Viracept HIV
Nembutal **PENTOBARBITAL** sedative, barbiturate
Neodecadron **NEOMYCIN & DEXAMETHASONE** antibiotic/steroid
NEOMYCIN Myciguent antibiotic
Neoral **CYCLOSPORINE** immunosuppressant
NEOSTIGMINE Prostigmin anticholinesterase
Neptazane **METHAZOLAMIDE** antiglaucoma
Neumega **OPRELVEKIN** thrombocytopenia
Neupogen **FILGRASTIM** anti-inflammatory
Neuramate **MEPROBAMATE** sedative, antianxiety
Neurontin **GABAPENTIN** anticonvulsant
NeuTrexin **TRIMETREXATE** antineoplastic
NEVIRAPINE Viramune HIV
Nexium **ESOMEPRAZOLE** gastric reflux
NIACIN Vitamin B_3 reduces cholesterol
Niacor **NIACIN** reduces cholesterol
NICARDIPINE Cardene antianginal, calcium channel blocker
NICOTINIC ACID NIACIN reduces cholesterol
NIFEDIPINE Procardia, Adalat antianginal, calcium channel blocker
Nilandron **NILUTAMIDE** prostate cancer
NILUTAMIDE Nilandron prostate cancer
NIMODIPINE Nimotop calcium channel blocker

Nimotop **NIMODIPINE** calcium channel blocker
Nipent **PENTOSTATIN** leukemia
NISOLDIPINE Sular hypertension
NITROFURANTOIN Macrodantin antibiotic
NITROGLYCERIN vasodilator, angina
Nitropress **NITROPRUSSIDE** antihypertensive
NITROPRUSSIDE Nitropress antihypertensive
Nix **PERMETHRIN** lice
NIZATIDINE Axid antiulcer
Nizoral **KETOCONAZOLE** antifungal
Nolvadex **TAMOXIFEN** breast cancer
Norco **HYDROCODONE** narcotic
Norcuron **VECURONIUM** neuromuscular blocker
Norditropin **SOMATROPIN** growth hormone
NOREPINEPHRINE Levophed hypotension
NORETHINDRONE Camila oral contraceptive
Norflex **ORPHENADRINE** muscle relaxant
NORFLOXACIN Noroxin antibiotic
Norgesic **ORPHENADRINE** analgesic
Normodyne **LABETALOL** β-blocker
Noroxin **NORFLOXACIN** antibiotic
Norpace **DISOPYRAMIDE** antiarrhythmic
Norpramin **DESIPRAMINE** tricyclic antidepressant
NORTRIPTYLINE Aventyl, Pamelor tricyclic
    antidepressant
Norvasc **AMLODIPINE** calcium channel blocker
Norvir **RITONAVIR** anti-infective
Novantrone **MITOXANTRONE** prostate cancer
Novolin **INSULIN** diabetes
Novolog **INSULIN** diabetes
NYSTATIN Mycostatin antifungal
Nubain **NALBUPHINE** narcotic
Numorphan **OXYMORPHINE** narcotic
Nuprin **IBUPROFEN** NSAID
NYSTATIN Mycostatin antifungal

Obenix **PHENTERMINE** appetite suppressant
Obezine **PHENDIMETRAZINE** appetite suppressant
OCTEOTIDE Sandostatin antidiarrheal
Octamide **METOCLOPRAMIDE** nausea
Ocufen **FLURBIPROFEN** NSAID
Ocupress **CARTEOLOL** β-blocker
OFLOXACIN Floxin antibiotic
Ogen **ESTROPIPATE** hormone
OLANZAPINE Zydis, Zyprexa schizophrenia
OLMESARTAN Benicar hypertension
OLSALAZINE Dipentum GI anti-inflammatory
OMEPRAZOLE PriLosec antiulcer
Omnicef **CEFDINIR** antibiotic
Omnipen **AMPICILLIN** antibiotic
Oncaspar **PEGASPARGASE** antineoplastic
ONDANSETRON Zofran antinausea
OPRELVEKIN Neumega thrombocytopenia
Opticrom **CROMOLYN** antiasthmatic, antiallergy
Orap **PIMOZIDE** chronic schizophrenia
Oretic **HYDROCHLOROTHIAZIDE** antihypertensive
Orinase **TOLBUTAMIDE** oral hypoglycemic agent
ORLISTAT Xenical obesity
ORPHENADRINE Norflex muscle relaxant
Orudis **KETOPROFEN** NSAID
Oruvail **KETOPROFEN** NSAID
OSELTAMIVIR Tamiflu antiviral
Osteocalcin **CALCITONIN** osteoporosis
Ovide **MALATHION** lice
Ovidrel **CHORIONIC GONADOTROPIN** ovulation
    stimulator
OXACILLIN Bactocill antibiotic
OXALIPLATIN Eloxatin oncology
OXAPROZIN Daypro NSAID
OXAZEPAM Serax sedative, benzodiazepine
OXCARBAZEPINE Trileptal anticonvulsant
OXICONAZOLE Oxistat NSAID

Oxistat **OXICONAZOLE** NSAID
OXTRIPHYLLINE Choledyl SA bronchodilator
OXYBUTYNIN CHLORIDE Ditropan overactive
  bladder
OXYCODONE Percolone narcotic
OxyContin **OXYCODONE** narcotic
OXYMORPHINE Numorphan narcotic
Oxy-R **OXYCODONE** narcotic
OXYTETRACYCLINE Terramycin antibiotic
OXYTOCIN Pitocin hormone, oxytocic

Pacerone **AMIODARONE** antiarrhythmic
PACLITAXEL Taxol oncology
PALIVIZUMAB Synagis antiviral RSV
PALONOSETRON Aloxi antiemetic
Pamelor **NORTRIPTYLINE** tricyclic antidepressant
PAMIDRONATE Aredia electrolyte modifier
PANCURONIUM Pavulon neuromuscular blocker
Panmycin **TETRACYCLINE** antibiotic
Panretin **ALITRETINOIN** oncology
PANTOPRAZOLE Protonix GI reflux
Panwarfin **WARFARIN** anticoagulant
Paraflex **CHLORZOXAZONE** muscle relaxant
Parafon Forte **CHLORZOXAZONE** muscle relaxant
PAREGORIC antidiarrheal
PARICALCITOL Zemplar hyperparathyroidism
Parlodel **BROMOCRIPTINE** anti-Parkinson's
PAROXETINE Paxil antidepressant
Patanol **OLOPATADINE** antihistamine
Pathocil **DICLOXACILLIN** antibiotic
Pavulon **PANCURONIUM** neuromuscular blocker
Paxil **PAROXETINE** antidepressant
Paxipam **HALAZEPAM** sedative, benzodiazepine
Pediazole **ERYTHROMYCIN** antibiotic
Peganone **ETHOTOIN** anticonvulsant
PEGASPARGASE Oncaspar antineoplastic

PEMOLINE Cylert CNS stimulant
PENBUTOLOL Levatol antihypertensive, β-blocker
PENCICLOVIR Denavir antiviral
Penetrex **ENOXACIN** anti-infective
PENICILLAMINE Cuprimine, Depen
    anti-inflammatory
Pentacarinate **PENTAMIDINE** anti-infective
PENTAMIDINE Pentacarinate anti-infective
Pentasa **MESALAMINE** Crohn's disease
PENTAZOCINE Talwin narcotic
PENTOBARBITAL Nembutal sedative, barbiturate
PENTOSAN POLYSULFATE Elmiron anti-inflammatory
PENTOSTATIN Nipent leukemia, anti-inflammatory
Pentothal **THIOPENTAL** anesthetic, anticonvulsant
PENTOXIFYLLINE Trental hemorrheologic agent
Pepcid **FAMOTIDINE** antiulcer
Percocet **ACETAMINOPHEN & OXYCODONE**
    narcotic analgesic
Percolone **OXYCODONE** narcotic
PERGOLIDE Permax anti-Parkinson's agent
Pergonal **MENOTROPINS** hormone
PERINDOPRIL Aceon antihypertensive
Periostat **DOXYCYCLINE** antibiotic
Permax **PERGOLIDE** anti-Parkinson's agent
PERMETHRIN Nix lice
PERPHENAZINE Trilafon antipsychotic, antiemetic
Persantin **DIPYRIDAMOLE** antiplatelet agent
PHENAZOPYRIDINE Pyridium urinary tract analgesic
Phendiet **PHENDIMETRAZINE** appetite suppressant
PHENDIMETRAZINE Adipost, Bontril appetite
    suppressant
Phendry **DIPHENHYDRAMINE** antihistamine
PHENELZINE SULFATE Nardil antidepressant
Phenergan **PROMETHAZINE** antiemetic, sedative
Pheneturide **PHENTERMINE** appetite suppressant
PHENOBARBITAL Donnatal sedative, barbiturate

PHENOTHIAZINE Largactil antipsychotic
PHENOXYBENZAMINE Dibenzyline antihypertensive
Phentercot **PHENTERMINE** appetite suppressant
PHENTERMINE Adipex-P, Zantryl appetite
    suppressant
PHENYTOIN Dilantin anticonvulsant
Photofrin **PORFIMER SODIUM** oncology
Phyllocontin **AMINOPHYLLINE** bronchodilator
PHYTONADIONE AquaMEPHYTOIN vitamin K
PILOCARPINE Adsorbocarpine antiglaucoma
PIMOZIDE Orap chronic schizophrenia
PINDOLOL Visken antihypertensive, β-blocker
PIOGLITAZONE Actos type II diabetes
PIPERACILLIN Pipracil antibiotic
Pipracil **PIPERACILLIN** antibiotic
PIRBUTEROL Maxair bronchodilator
PIROXICAM Feldene NSAID
Pitocin **OXYTOCIN** hormone, oxytocic
Pitressin **VASOPRESSIN** hormone-antidiuretic
Placidyl **ETHCHLORVYNOL** sedative
Platinol **CISPLATIN** oncology
Plavix **CLOPIDROGREL** antiplatelet agent
Plegine **PHENDIMETRAZINE** appetite suppressant
Plendil **FELODIPINE** calcium channel blocker,
    antihypertensive
Pletal **CILOSTAZOL** intermittent claudication
PLICAMYCIN Mithracin, Mithramycin antineoplastic
PMB 200 **PREMARIN & MEPROBAMATE**
    menopause, antianxiety
PODOFILOX Condylox genital warts
Polycillin **AMPICILLIN** antibiotic
POLYETHYLENE GLYCOL Golytely constipation
POLYMYXIN B Aerosporin antibiotic
Polymyxin E **COLISTIN** antibiotic
POLYTHIAZIDE Renese diuretic
Ponstel **MEFENAMIC ACID** NSAID

PORFIMER SODIUM Photofrin oncology
PRAMIPEXOLE Mirapex Parkinson's disease
Prandin **REPAGLINIDE** diabetes
Pravachol **PRAVASTATIN** lipid-lowering agent
PRAVASTATIN Pravachol lipid-lowering agent
PRAZEPAM Centrax sedative, benzodiazepine
PRAZOSIN Minipress antihypertensive
PRAZOSIN & POLYTHIAZIDE Minizide hypertension
Precose **ACARBOSE** hypoglycemia
PREDNISOLONE Prelone anti-inflammatory
PREDNISONE Deltasone corticosteroid
Prehist **CHLORPHENIRAMINE & PHENYLEPHRINE**
    antihistamine-decongestant
Prelone **PREDNISOLONE** anti-inflammatory
Prelu-2 **PHENDIMETRAZINE** appetite suppressant
Premarin **ESTROGEN** hormone
Prevacid **LANSOPRAZOLE** antiulcer agent
Prevpac **LANSOPRAZOLE** antiulcer agent
Priften **RIFAPENTINE** anti-infective
PriLosec **OMEPRAZOLE** antiulcer
Primacor **MILRINONE** inotropic/vasodilator agent
Primaxin **IMIPENEM** antibiotic
PRIMIDONE Mysoline anticonvulsant
Prinivil **LISINOPRIL** ACE inhibitor
Prinzide **LISINOPRIL & HCTZ** antihypertensive
Priscoline **TOLAZOLINE** antihypertensive
ProAmatine **MIDODRINE** orthostatic hypotension
Probate **MEPROBAMATE** sedative, antianxiety
Pro-Banthine **PROPANTHELINE** anticholinergic
PROBENECID Benemid antigout
PROCAINAMIDE Pronestyl antiarrhythmic
Procan **PROCAINAMIDE** antiarrhythmic
Procardia **NIFEDIPINE** antianginal, calcium channel
    blocker
PROCHLORPERAZINE Compazine antiemetic
PROCYCLIDINE Kemadrin Parkinson's

Pro-Fast **PHENTERMINE** appetite suppressant
Prograf **TACROLIMUS** immunosuppressant
Prolixin **FLUPHENAZINE** antipsychotic, phenothiazine
Proloprim **TRIMETHOPRIM** UTI, antibiotic
PROMAZINE Sparine antipsychotic
Prometa **METAPROTERENOL** anti-asthmatic
PROMETHAZINE Anergan, Phenergan antiemetic
Promine **PROCAINAMIDE** antiarrhythmic
Pronestyl **PROCAINAMIDE** antiarrhythmic
PROPAFENONE Rhythmol antiarrhythmic
PROPANTHELINE Pro-Banthine anticholinergic
Propecia **FINASTERIDE** hair growth
PROPOXYPHENE Darvon narcotic
Propulsid **CISAPRIDE** anti-GI reflux agent
PROPRANOLOL Inderal, Inderide β-blocker
PROPYLTHIOURACIL PTU antithyroid agent
Proscar **FINASTERIDE** enzyme inhibitor
ProSom **ESTAZOLAM** sedative, benzodiazepine
Prostigmin **NEOSTIGMINE** anticholinesterase
Protonix **PANTOPRAZOLE** GI reflux
Protostat **METRONIDAZOLE** Crohn's disease
PROTRIPTYLINE Vivactil tricyclic antidepressant
Proventil **ALBUTEROL** bronchodilator
Provera **MEDROXYPROGESTERONE** oncology
Provigil **MODAFINIL** narcolepsy
Prozac **FLUOXETINE** antidepressant
PSEUDOEPHEDRINE Sudafed decongestant
Psorcon **DIFLORASONE** steroid
PSYLLIUM Hydrocil constipation
PT 105 **PHENDIMETRAZINE** appetite suppressant
PTU **PROPYLTHIOURACIL** antithyroid agent
Pulvules **CINOXACIN** antibiotic
Pulmicort **BUDESONIDE** asthma, steroid
Pulmozyme **DORNASE ALFA** mucolytic
PYRAZINAMIDE Rifator anti-infective
PYRIDOSTIGMINE Mestinon myasthenia gravis

Pyridium **PHENAZOPYRIDINE** urinary tract analgesic
PYRIMETHAMINE Daraprim malaria
PYRIDOSTIGMINE Regonol cholinergic

Quadramet **SAMARIUM** oncology
QUAZEPAM Doral benzodiazepine
Questran **CHOLESTYRAMINE** antilipemic
QUETIAPINE Seroquel psychosis
Quibron **GUAIFENESIN & THEOPHYLLINE**
  bronchodilator
QUINAPRIL Accupril ACE inhibitor
Quinaretic **QUINAPRIL & HCTZ** ACE inhibitor
Quinidex **QUINIDINE** antiarrhythmic
QUINIDINE Quinidex antiarrhythmic
QUININE antimalarial
Qvar **BETACLOMETHASONE** asthma

RABEPRAZOLE AcipHex gastric acid inhibitor
RALOXIFENE E-Vista osteoporosis
RAMIPRIL Altace antihypertensive, ACE inhibitor
RANITIDINE Zantac antiulcer
Rapamune **SIROLIMUS** immunosuppressant
RASBURICASE Elitek uric acid reducer
Raxar **GREPAFLOXACIN** anti-infective
Rebetrol **RIBAVIRIN** Hepatitis C
Rebif **INTERFERON BETA 1a** antiviral
Reyataz **ATAZANAVIR** HIV
Reglan **METOCLOPRAMIDE** antiemetic, GI stimulant
Regonol **PYRIDOSTIGMINE** cholinergic
Relafen **NABUMETONE** NSAID
Relenza **ZANAMIVIR** antiviral
Relpax **ELETRIPTAN** migraine
Remeron **MIRTAZAPINE** depression
Remicade **INFLIXIMAB** Crohn's disease
Reminyl **GALANTAMINE** Alzheimer's
Renagel **SEVELAMER** phosphate binder

Renese **POLYTHIAZIDE** diuretic
REPAGLINIDE Prandin diabetes
Repronex **MENOTROPINS** fertility drug
Requip **ROPINIROLE** anti-Parkinson's
RESERPINE Serpalan antihypertensive
Rescriptor **DELAVIRDINE** antiviral
Restasis **CYCLOSPORIN** immunosuppressant
Restoril **TEMAZEPAM** sedative, benzodiazepine
Retavase **RETEPLASE** acute MI, pulmonary embolism
RETEPLASE Retavase acute MI, pulmonary embolism
Retin-A **TRETINOIN** endocrine
Retrovir **AZT ZIDOVUDINE** antiviral
Revex **NALMEFENE** narcotic antagonist
Reyataz **ATAZANAVIR** antiviral
Rheumatrex **METHOTREXATE** anti-inflammatory
Rhinocart **BUDESONIDE** glucocorticoid
RIBAVIRIN Rebetrol Hepatitis C
Ridaura **AURANOFIN** anti-inflammatory
Rifadin **RIFAMPIN** antibiotic
Rifamate **RIFAMPIN & ISONIAZID** tuberculosis
RIFAMPIN Rifadin antibiotic
RIFAPENTINE Priften anti-infective
Rifator **PYRAZINAMIDE** anti-infective
Rilutek **RILUZOLE** amyotrophic lateral sclerosis
RILUZOLE Rilutek amyotrophic lateral sclerosis
Rimactane **RIFAMPIN** antibiotic
RIMANTADINE Flumadine antiviral
RIMEXOLONE Vexol corticosteroid
RISEDRONATE Actonel Paget's disease, osteoporosis
Risperdal **RISPERIDONE** antipsychotic
RISPERIDONE Risperdal antipsychotic
Ritalin **METHYLPHENIDATE** CNS stimulant
RITONAVIR Norvir anti-infective
Rituxin **RITUXIMAB** oncology
RITUXIMAB Rituxin oncology
RIVASTIGMINE Exelon Alzheimer's

RIZATRIPTAN Maxalt migraine
Robaxin **METHOCARBAMOL** skeletal muscle relaxant
Robinul **GLYCOPYRROLATE** peptic ulcers
Rocephin **CEFTRIAXONE** antibiotic
ROCURONIUM Zemuron neuromuscular blocking
   agent
ROFECOXIB Vioxx anti-inflammatory
Rogaine **MINOXIDIL** hair-growing agent
Romazicon **FLUMAZENIL** benzodiazepine antagonist
Rondec **CARBINOXAMINE** antihistamine
ROPINIROLE Requip anti-Parkinson's
ROSIGLITAZONE Avandia diabetes
Rowasa **MESALAMINE** Crohn's disease
Roxicet **OXYCODONE & ACETAMINOPHEN** analgesic
Roxicodone **OXYCODONE** analgesic
Rynatuss **CARBETAPENTANE** cough
Rythmol **PROPAFENONE** antiarrhythmic

SACROSIDASE Sucraid enzyme replacement
SALMETEROL Serevent bronchodilator
SALMETEROL & FLUTICASONE Advair DisKus steroid
Salofalk **MESALAMINE** Crohn's disease
SALSALATE Mono-Gesic NSAID, antipyretic
Saluron **HYDROFLUMETHIAZIDE** diuretic
SAMARIUM Quadramet oncology
Sandimmune **CYCLOSPORINE** immunosuppressant
Sandostatin **OCTEOTIDE** antidiarrheal
Sanorex **MAZINDOL** obesity
Sansert **METHYSERGIDE** vascular headache
SAQUINAVIR Invirase anti-infective
Sarafem **FLUOXETINE** antidepressant
SCOPOLAMINE antiemetic
SECOBARBITAL Seconal sedative, barbiturate
Seconal **SECOBARBITAL** sedative, barbiturate
Sectral **ACEBUTOLOL** antihypertensive

Sedapap **BUTALBITAL & ACETAMINOPHEN** tension headache

Seldane **TERFENADINE** antihistamine

SELEGILINE Eldepryl, Atapryl anti-Parkinson's

Semprex-D **ACRIVASTINE & PSEUDOEPHEDRINE** antihistamine-decongestant

SENNA Senokot laxative

Senokot **SENNA** laxative

Septra **TRIMETHOPRIM & SULFAMETHOXAZOLE** antibiotic

Serax **OXAZEPAM** sedative, benzodiazepine

Serentil **MESORIDAZINE** antipsychotic

Serevent **SALMETEROL** bronchodilator

Serlect **SERTINDOLE** schizophrenia

Serophene **CLOMIPHENE** hormone

Serostim **SOMATROPIN** growth hormone

Seroquel **QUETIAPINE** psychosis

Serpalan **RESERPINE** antihypertensive

SERTINDOLE Serlect schizophrenia

SERTRALINE Zoloft antidepressant

Serzone **NEFAZODONE** antidepressant

SEVELAMER Renagel phosphate binder

SIBUTRAMINE Meridia obesity

SILDENAFIL Viagra erectile dysfunction

SIMVASTATIN Zocor lipid-lowering agent

Sinaquan **DOXEPIN** tricyclic antidepressant

Sinemet **CARBIDOPA & LEVODOPA** Parkinson's

Singulair **MONTELUKAST** antiallergic

SIROLIMUS Rapamune immunosuppressant

Skelaxin **METAXALONE** muscle relaxant

Slo-bid **THEOPHYLLINE** bronchodilator

Solu-Cortef **HYDROCORTISONE** glucocorticoid, short-acting

Solu-Medrol **METHYLPREDNISOLONE** steroid

Soma **CARISOPRODOL** muscle relaxant

SOMATROPIN Humatrope growth hormone

Somophyllin **AMINOPHYLLINE** bronchodilator
Sonata **ZALEPLON** hypnotic
Soriatane **ACITRETIN** severe psoriasis
SOTALOL Betapace β-blocker
SPARFLOXACIN Zagam pneumonia
Sparine **PROMAZINE** antipsychotic
Spectazole **ECONAZOLE** antifungal
SPECTINOMYCIN Trobicin antibiotic
Spectracef **CEFDITOREN** antibiotic
Spectrobid **BACAMPICILLIN** antibiotic
SPIRONOLACTONE Aldactone diuretic
Sporanox **ITRACONAZOLE** anti-infective
Stadol **BUTORPHANOL** narcotic
Stagesic **HYDROCODONE & ACETAMINOPHEN**
    analgesic
Staphcillin **METHICILLIN** antibiotic
STAVUDINE Zerit antiviral
Stelazine **TRIFLUOPERAZINE** sedative
Strattera **ATOMOXETINE** ADHD
STREPTOKINASE thrombolytic
STREPTOMYCIN antibiotic
Stromectol **IVERMECTIN** anti-parasite
STRONTIUM-89 CHLORIDE Metastron analgesic
Sublimaze **FENTANYL** narcotic analgesic
Suboxone **BUPRENORPHINE & NALOXONE**
    treatment of opioid addiction
Subutex **BUPRENORPHINE** narcotic
SUCCINYLCHOLINE Anectine neuromuscular
    blocker
Sucraid **SCROSIDASE** enzyme replacement
SUCRALFATE Carafate antiulcer
Sudafed **PSEUDOEPHEDRINE** decongestant
Sufenta **SUFENTANIL** narcotic
SUFENTANIL Sufenta narcotic
Sular **NISOLDIPINE** hypertension
SULFACETAMIDE Cetamide antifungal

SULFAMETHOXAZOLE Septra antibiotic
SULFASALAZINE Azulfidine antibiotic
SULFISOXAZOLE Gantrisin, Pediazole antibiotic
SULINDAC Clinoril NSAID
SUMATRIPTAN Imitrex migraine
Suprax **CEFIXIME** antibiotic
Surmontil **TRIMIPRAMINE** tricyclic antidepressant
Sustiva **EFAVIRENZ** antiviral
Symadine **AMANTADINE** anti-Parkinson's
Symbyax **OLANZAPINE & FLUOXETINE** treatment
    of bipolar disorder
Symmetrel **AMANTADINE** anti-Parkinson
Synagis **PALIVIZUMAB** antiviral RSV
Synalgos **DIHYDROCODEINE** narcotic
Synarel **NAFARELIN** hormone
Synthroid **LEVOTHYROXINE** thyroid

Tabloid **THIOGUANINE** leukemia
Tace **CHLOROTRIANISENE** estrogen
TACRINE Cognex Alzheimer's dementia
TACROLIMUS Prograf immunosuppressant
Tagamet **CIMETIDINE** antiulcer
Talwin **PENTAZOCINE** narcotic
Tambocor **FLECAINIDE** antiarrhythmic
Tamiflu **OSELTAMIVIR** antiviral
TAMOXIFEN Nolvadex breast cancer
TAMSULOSIN Flomax prostatic hyperplasia
Tao **TROLEANDOMYCIN** antibiotic
Tapazole **METHIMAZOLE** antithyroid agent
Tarka **TRANDOLAPRIL & VERAPAMIL**
    ACE inhibitor-calcium channel blocker
Tasmar **TOLCAPONE** Parkinson's
Tavist **CLEMASTINE** antihistamine
Taxol **PACLITAXEL** oncology
Tazidime **CEFTAZIDIME** antibiotic
TEGASEROD Zelnorm constipation

Tegretol **CARBAMAZEPINE** anticonvulsant
TELITHROMYCIN Ketek antibiotic
TELMISARTAN Micardis hypertension
TEMAZEPAM Restoril sedative, benzodiazepine
Tenex **GUANFACINE** antihypertensive
Tenormin **ATENOLOL** antihypertensive, β-blocker
Tensilon **EDROPHONIUM** cholinergic-
    anti-cholinesterase
Tenuate **DIETHYLPROPION** obesity
Tequin **GATIFLOXACIN** antibiotic
TERAZOSIN Hytrin antihypertensive
TERBINAFINE Lamisil anti-infective
TERBUTALINE Brethaire, Brethine bronchodilator
TERFENADINE Seldane antihistamine
TERIPARATIDE Forteo osteoporosis
Terramycin **OXYTETRACYCLINE** antibiotic
Tessalon **BENZONATATE** antitussive
TETRACYCLINE antibiotic
Teveten **EPROSARTAN** hypertension
Theo-Dur **THEOPHYLLINE** bronchodilator
Theolair **THEOPHYLLINE** bronchodilator
THEOPHYLLINE Aerolate, Slo-bid, Theo-Dur
    bronchodilator
THIABENDAZOLE Mintezol antiparasitic
THIETHYLPERAZINE Torecan antiemetic
THIOGUANINE Lanvis oncology
Thiola **TIOPRONIN** kidney stone prevention
THIOPENTAL Pentothal anesthetic, anticonvulsant
THIORIDAZINE Mellaril antipsychotic
THIOTHIXENE Navane antipsychotic
Thorazine **CHLORPROMAZINE** antipsychotic
Thyrolar **LIOTRIX** thyroid
TIAGABINE Gabitril epilepsy
Tiazac **DILTIAZEM** calcium channel blocker
Ticar **TICARCILLIN** antibiotic
TICARCILLIN Ticar antibiotic

Ticlid **TICLOPIDINE** cardiovascular
TICLOPIDINE Ticlid cardiovascular
Tigan **TRIMETHOBENZAMIDE** antiemetic
Tikosyn **DOFETILIDE** antiarrhythmic
Tilade **NEDOCROMIL** mast cell stabilizer
Timentin **TICARCILLIN & CLAVULANATE** antibiotic
Timolide **TIMOLOL & HCTZ** β-blocker-diuretic
TIMOLOL Blocadren β-blocker
TIOPRONIN Thiola kidney stone prevention
TIROFIBAN Aggrastat unstable angina
TIZANIDINE Zanaflex neurologic
TOBRAMYCIN Tobrex antibiotic
Tobrex **TOBRAMYCIN** antibiotic
TOCAINIDE Tonocard antiarrhythmic
Tofranil **IMIPRAMINE** tricyclic antidepressant
TOLAZAMIDE Tolinase oral hypoglycemic agent
TOLAZOLINE Priscoline antihypertensive
TOLBUTAMIDE Orinase oral hypoglycemic agent
TOLCAPONE Tasmar Parkinson's
Tolectin **TOLMETIN** NSAID
Tolinase **TOLAZAMIDE** oral hypoglycemic agent
TOLMETIN Tolectin NSAID
TOLTERODINE Detrol overactive bladder
Tonocard **TOCAINIDE** antiarrhythmic
Topamax **TOPIRAMATE** neurologic
TOPIRAMATE Topamax neurologic
TOPOTECAN Hycamtin oncology
Toprol **METOPROLOL** β-blocker
Toradol **KETOROLAC** NSAID, non-narcotic analgesic
Torecan **THIETHYLPERAZINE** antiemetic
TOREMIFENE Fareston oncology
Tornalate **BITOLTEROL** bronchodilator, asthma
TORSEMIDE Demadex diuretic
Tracrium **ATRACURIUM** neuromuscular blocking
    agent
TRAMADOL Ultram analgesic

Tracleer **BOSENTAN** pulmonary hypertension
Trancopal **CHLORMEZANONE** antianxiety agent
Trandate **LABETALOL** antihypertensive
TRANDOLAPRIL Mavik hypertension
Tranxene **CLORAZEPATE** antianxiety agent
TRASTUZUMAB Herceptin oncology
TRAZODONE Desyrel antidepressant
Trelstar Depot **TRIPTORELIN** oncology
Trental **PENTOXIFYLLINE** hemorrheologic agent
TRETINOIN Avita, Retin-A acne
Trexall **METHOTREXATE** oncology
TRIAMCINOLONE Azmacort steroid, asthma
TRIAMTERENE Dyrenium diuretic
Triavil **PERPHENAZINE & AMITRIPTYLINE**
    antidepressant
TRIAZOLAM Halcion sedative, benzodiazepine
TRICHLORMETHIAZIDE Metahydrin diuretic
Tricor **FENOFIBRATE** antilipemic
Tridione **TRIMETHADIONE** antiepileptic
TRIFLUOPERAZINE Stelazine sedative
TRIHEXYPHENIDYL Artane anti-Parkinson's
Trilafon **PERPHENAZINE** antipsychotic, antiemetic
Trileptal **OXCARBAZEPINE** anticonvulsant
Trilisate **CHOLINE MAGNESIUM TRISALICYLATE**
    non-narcotic analgesic
TRIMETHADIONE Tridione antiepileptic
TRIMETHAPHAN Arfonad antihypertensive
TRIMETHOBENZAMIDE Tigan antiemetic
TRIMETHOPRIM Proloprim UTI, antibiotic
TRIMETREXATE NeuTrexin antineoplastic
TRIMIPRAMINE Surmontil tricyclic antidepressant
Trimox **AMOXICILLIN** antibiotic
TRIPTORELIN Trelstar Depot oncology
Trisenox **ARSENIC** leukemia
Trizivir **ABACAVIR/LAMIVUDINE/ZIDOVUDINE**
    antiviral

Trobicin **SPECTINOMYCIN** antibiotic
TROLEANDOMYCIN Tao antibiotic
TROVAFLOXACIN Trovan antibiotic
Trovan **TROVAFLOXACIN** antibiotic
Trusopt **DORZOLAMIDE** glaucoma
Tylenol **ACETAMINOPHEN** antipyretic, analgesic

Ultrabrom **BROMPHENIRAMINE &
    PSEUDOEPHEDRINE** antihistamine
Ultram **TRAMADOL** analgesic
Ultravate **HALOBETASOL** steroid
Uniretic **MOEXIPRIL** antihypertensive
Unisom **DOXYLAMINE** sedative
Univasc **MOEXIPRIL** antihypertensive
Urecholine **BETHANECHOL** urinary retention
Urex **METHENAMINE** antibiotic, UTI
Urispas **FLAVOXATE** bladder antispasmodic
Uroaxtral **ALFUZOSIN** muscle relaxer
UROFOLLITIN Fertinex induces ovulation
UROFOLLITROPIN Bravelle infertility
UROKINASE Abbokinase thrombolytic
URSODIOL Actigall dissolves gall stones

Vagifem **ESTRADIOL** hormone
VALACYCLOVIR Valtrex herpes zoster
VALDECOXIB Bextra NSAID
Valium **DIAZEPAM** benzodiazepine, sedative
VALPROIC ACID Depakene anticonvulsant
Valrelease **DIAZEPAM** benzodiazepine, sedative
VALSARTAN Diovan hypertension
Valtrex **VALACYCLOVIR** herpes zoster
Vanatrip **AMITRIPTYLINE** tricyclic antidepressant
Vancenase **BECLOMETHASONE** steroid, asthma
Vanceril **BETACLOMETHASONE** asthma
Vancocin **VANCOMYCIN** antibiotic
VANCOMYCIN Vancocin antibiotic

Vaniqa **EFLORNITHINE** hair growth inhibitor

Vantin **CEFPODOXIME PROXETIL** antibiotic

VARENICLINE Chantix smoking cessation

VARDENAFIL Levitra erectile dysfunction

Vascor **BEPRIDIL** calcium channel blocker

Vaserectic **ENALAPRIL MALEATE & HYDROCHLOROTHIAZIDE** antihypertensive

VASOPRESSIN Pitressin hormone-antidiuretic

Vasotec **ENALAPRIL** antihypertensive

Vectrin **MINOCYCLINE** antibiotic

VECURONIUM Norcuron neuromuscular blocker

Velosef **CEPHRADINE** antibiotic

VENLAFAXINE Effexor antidepressant

Ventolin **ALBUTEROL** bronchodilator

VERAPAMIL Calan, Isoptin calcium channel blocker

Versed **MIDAZOLAM** sedative, benzodiazepine

Vexol **RIMEXOLONE** corticosteroid

Viagra **SILDENAFIL** erectile dysfunction

Vibramycin **DOXYCYCLINE** antibiotic

Vicodin **ACETAMINOPHEN & HYDROCODONE** narcotic analgesic

Vicoprofen **HYDROCODONE & IBUPROFEN** narcotic analgesic, NSAID

VIDARABINE Vira-A antiviral

Videx **DIDANOSINE** antiviral

VINORELBINE Navelbine antineoplastic

Vioxx **ROFECOXIB** anti-inflammatory

Vira-A **VIDARABINE** antiviral

Viracept **NELFINAVIR** HIV

Viramune **NEVIRAPINE** HIV

Visken **PINDOLOL** antihypertensive, β-blocker

Vistaject **HYDROXYZINE** sedative

Vistaril **HYDROXYZINE** sedative

Vitrasert **GANCICLOVIR** antiviral

Vivactil **PROTRIPTYLINE** tricyclic antidepressant

Vivelle **ESTRADIOL** hormone

Volmax **ALBUTEROL** bronchodilator
Voltaren **DICLOFENAC** NSAID

WARFARIN Coumadin anticoagulant
WelChol **COLESEVELAM** anti-lipemic
Wellbutrin **BUPROPION** antidepressant
Wigraine **ERGOTAMINE** migraine
Wygesic **PROPOXYPHENE & ACETAMINOPHEN**
 pain control
Wytensin **GUANABENZ** antihypertensive

Xalaton **LATANOPROST** glaucoma
Xanax **ALPRAZOLAM** sedative, benzodiazepine
Xeloda **CAPECITABINE** oncology
Xenical **ORLISTAT** obesity
Xigris **DROTRECOGIN ALFA** sepsis
Xopenex **LEVALBUTEROL** asthma

Zaditor **KETOTIFEN** antihistamine
ZAFIRLUKAST Accolate inhibits bronchospasm
Zagam **SPARFLOXACIN** pneumonia
ZALCITABINE Hivid anti-infective
ZALEPLON Sonata hypnotic
Zanaflex **TIZANIDINE** neurologic
ZANAMIVIR Relenza antiviral
Zantac **RANITIDINE** antiulcer
Zantryl **PHENTERMINE HCL** appetite suppressant
Zarontin **ETHOSUXIMIDE** anticonvulsant
Zaroxolyn **METOLAZONE** diuretic, antihypertensive
Zebeta **BISOPROLOL** β-blocker, antihypertensive
Zefazone **CEFMETAZOLE** antibiotic
Zelnorm **TEGASEROD** constipation
Zemplar **PARICALCITOL** hyperparathyroidism
Zemuron **ROCURONIUM** neuromuscular blocking
 agent
Zerit **STAVUDINE** antiviral

Zestril **LISINOPRIL** ACE inhibitor
Zetia **EZETIMIBE** anti-lipemic
Ziagen **ABACAVIR** anti-infective, HIV
Ziac **BISOPROLOL & HYDROCHLOROTHIAZIDE**
    antihypertensive, β-blocker
ZIDOVUDINE AZT antiviral
ZILEUTON Zyflo asthma
Zithromax **AZITHROMYCIN** antibiotic
ZIPRASIDONE Geodon schizophrenia
Zocor **SIMVASTATIN** cholesterol-lowering agent
Zofran **ONDANSETRON** antiemetic
Zoladex **GOSERELIN ACETATE** oncology
ZOLMITRIPTAN Zomig migraine
Zoloft **SERTRALINE** antidepressant
ZOLPIDEM Ambien insomnia
Zomig **ZOLMITRIPTAN** migraine
Zonegran **ZONISAMIDE** seizures
ZONISAMIDE Zonegran seizures
Zovia **ETHYNODIOL DIACETATE & ETHINYL**
    ESTRADIOL oral contraceptive
Zyban **BUPROPION** antidepressant
Zydis **OLANZAPINE** psychotropic
Zyflo **ZILEUTON** asthma
Zyloprim **ALLOPURINOL** anti-gout
Zyprexa **OLANZAPINE** psychotropic
Zyrtec **CETIRIZINE** antihistamine
Zyvox **LINEZOLID** antibacterial

PALS

Bradycardia with Poor Perfusion

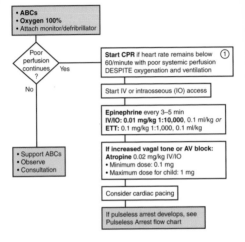

- ABCs
- Oxygen 100%
- Attach monitor/defibrillator

Poor perfusion continues?
Yes →

Start CPR if heart rate remains below 60/minute with poor systemic perfusion DESPITE oxygenation and ventilation ①

Start IV or intraosseous (IO) access

Epinephrine every 3–5 min
IV/IO: **0.01 mg/kg 1:10,000,** 0.1 ml/kg or
ETT: 0.1 mg/kg 1:1,000, 0.1 ml/kg

If increased vagal tone or AV block:
Atropine 0.02 mg/kg IV/IO
- Minimum dose: 0.1 mg
- Maximum dose for child: 1 mg

Consider cardiac pacing

If pulseless arrest develops, see Pulseless Arrest flow chart

No ↓

- Support ABCs
- Observe
- Consultation

CPR
- **When intubation complete:** rescuers no longer deliver "cycles" of CPR. Give continuous chest compressions without pauses for breaths. Give 8–10 breaths/minute. Check rhythm every 2 minutes.
- **Compressions:** 100/min, ensure full chest recoil, minimize interruptions.
- **One cycle = 15 compressions then 2 breaths.**
- **Do not interrupt CPR when giving medications.**

1 **During CPR:** attempt and verify tracheal intubation and start an IV. Identify and treat causes: hypotension, hypovolemia, hypothermia, electrolytes, tamponade, tension pneumothorax, toxins (overdose), thromboembolism. Be certain you are providing adequate oxygenation and ventilation.

Pulseless Arrest

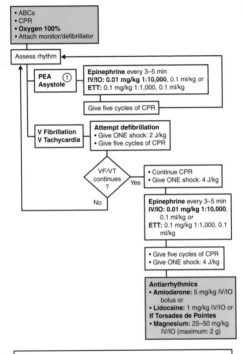

CPR
- **When intubation complete:** rescuers no longer deliver "cycles" of CPR. Give continuous chest compressions without pauses for breaths. Give 8–10 breaths/minute. Check rhythm every 2 minutes.
- **Compressions:** 100/min, ensure full chest recoil, minimize interruptions.
- **One cycle** = 15 compressions then 2 breaths.
- Do not interrupt CPR when giving medications.

1 **Search for causes:** hypovolemia, hypoxia, acidosis, hypokalemia, hypoglycemia, hypothermia, toxins, cardiac tamponade, tension pneumothorax, PE, trauma.

Tachycardia with Adequate Perfusion

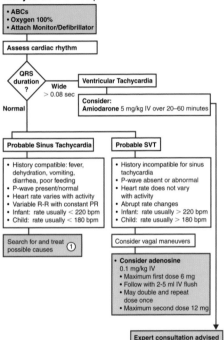

```
• ABCs
• Oxygen 100%
• Attach Monitor/Defibrillator
        │
Assess cardiac rhythm
        │
   ┌─────────┐
   │  QRS    │    Wide          Ventricular Tachycardia
   │ duration│──────> 0.08 sec
   │   ?     │                  Consider:
   └─────────┘                  Amiodarone 5 mg/kg IV over 20–60 minutes
        │
     Normal
```

Probable Sinus Tachycardia	Probable SVT
• History compatible: fever, dehydration, vomiting, diarrhea, poor feeding • P-wave present/normal • Heart rate varies with activity • Variable R-R with constant PR • Infant: rate usually < 220 bpm • Child: rate usually < 180 bpm	• History incompatible for sinus tachycardia • P-wave absent or abnormal • Heart rate does not vary with activity • Abrupt rate changes • Infant: rate usually > 220 bpm • Child: rate usually > 180 bpm

Search for and treat possible causes ①

Consider vagal maneuvers

• **Consider adenosine**
0.1 mg/kg IV
• Maximum first dose 6 mg
• Follow with 2-5 ml IV flush
• May double and repeat dose once
• Maximum second dose 12 mg

Expert consultation advised

1 Search for causes: hypovolemia, hypoxia, acidosis, hypokalemia, hypoglycemia, hypothermia, toxins, cardiac tamponade, tension pneumothorax, PE, trauma.

Tachycardia with Poor Perfusion

- ABCs
- Oxygen
- Monitor Cardiac Rhythm

Pulse present ? — **No** →
- Start CPR
- See **Pulseless Arrest** algorithm

Yes

QRS duration ? — **Wide** > 0.08 sec →

Normal

Probable VT

Immediate cardioversion
0.5–1 J/kg, then 2 J/kg ①

Probable Sinus Tachycardia

- History compatible: dehydration, fever, vomiting, diarrhea, poor feeding
- P-wave present/normal
- Heart rate varies with activity
- Variable R-R with constant PR
- Infant: rate usually < 220 bpm
- Child: rate usually < 180 bpm

Search for and treat possible causes ②

Probable SVT

- History incompatible for sinus tachycardia
- P-wave absent or abnormal
- Heart rate does not vary with activity
- History of abrupt rate changes
- Infant: rate usually ≥ 220 bpm
- Child: rate usually ≥ 180 bpm

Consider vagal maneuvers

- If IV access immediately available:
- **Adenosine** 0.1 mg/kg/ IV/IO rapid bolus
  - Maximum first dose 6 mg
  - Maximum second dose 12 mg
OR
- **Immediate cardioversion** 0.5–1 J/kg
  - May increase to 2 J/kg
  - Sedate if does not cause delay

- Expert consultation advised
- Consider **amiodarone** 5 mg/kg IV over 20–60 min

1   **Synchronized cardioversion:** may use **adenosine** and/or **sedation** prior to cardioversion, yet these efforts should not delay cardioversion.
2   **Search for causes:** hypovolemia, hypoxia, acidosis, hypokalemia, hypoglycemia, hypothermia, toxins, cardiac tamponade, tension pneumothorax, PE, trauma.

Basic Life Support

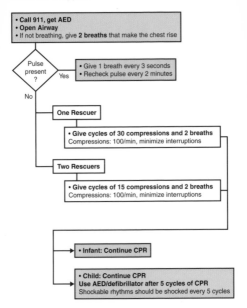

CPR • Child: Continue CPR, use AED after 5 cycles of CPR.
• **When intubation complete:** rescuers no longer deliver "cycles" of CPR. Give continuous chest compressions without pauses for breaths. Give 8–10 breaths/minute. Check rhythm every 2 minutes.
• **Compressions:** 100/min, ensure full chest recoil, minimize interruptions.

NRP

Neonatal Resuscitation

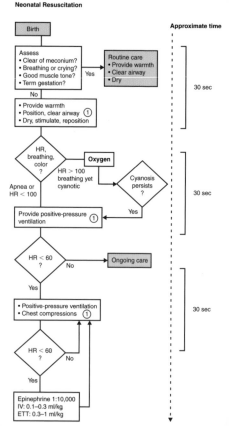

1 Endotracheal intubation may be considered at several steps.

Newborn Resuscitation

Assess and
support

Always needed

Needed less
frequently

Rarely needed

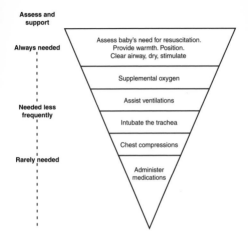

Assess baby's need for resuscitation.
Provide warmth. Position.
Clear airway, dry, stimulate

Supplemental oxygen

Assist ventilations

Intubate the trachea

Chest compressions

Administer
medications

Abbreviations

ABCs	airway, breathing, and circulation
ABG	arterial blood gas
AV	atrioventricular
BE	base excess
bid	twice a day
BP	blood pressure
BSA	body surface area
BUN	blood urea nitrogen
CHF	congestive heart failure
CO	cardiac output
DTaP	diphtheria, tetanus, and acellular pertussis (vaccine)
D5W	5% dextrose in water
EEG	electroencephalogram
EKG	electrocardiogram
ET	endotracheal
ETT	endotracheal tube
Fr	French (scale)
g	gram
GI	gastrointestinal
h	hour
HCO$_3$	bicarbonate
Hct	hematocrit
Hgb	hemoglobin
HR	heart rate
I&O	intake & output
ICP	intracranial pressure
IM	intramuscular
INR	international normalized ratio
IO	intraosseous
IV	intravenous

IVP	intravenous push
J	joule
KCL	potassium chloride
kg	kilogram
LOC	loss of consciousness
LR	lactated Ringer's (solution)
MAT	multifocal atrial tachycardia
mcg	microgram
mEq	milliequivalent
mg	milligram
ml	milliliter
MMR	measles, mumps, rubella (vaccine)
mo	month
N	nausea
N/V	nausea and/or vomiting
NG	nasogastric
NRP	Neonatal Resuscitation Program
NS	normal saline
Paco$_2$	partial pressure of carbon dioxide, arterial
PALS	pediatric advanced life support
Pao$_2$	partial pressure of oxygen, arterial
PAWP	pulmonary artery wedge pressure
PEA	pulseless electrical activity
PO	per mouth
PR	per rectum
prn	as needed
PSVT	paroxysmal supraventricular tachycardia
PTT	partial thromboplastin time
PVC	premature ventricular contraction
q	every
RBC	red blood cell
SA	sinoatrial
SC	subcutaneous

SL	sublingual
SOB	shortness of breath
SVT	supraventricular tachycardia
SW	sterile water
tid	three times a day
U	unit
V	vomiting
VF	ventricular fibrillation
VS	vital signs
VT	ventricular tachycardia
vWF	von Willebrand factor
WBC	white blood cell
WNL	within normal limits
y	year

Notes

_____

_____

_____

_____

_____

_____

_____

_____

_____

_____

_____

_____

_____

_____

_____

_____

_____

_____

_____

Notes

_____

_____

_____

_____

_____

_____

_____

_____

_____

_____

_____

_____

_____

_____

_____

_____

_____

_____

_____

Notes

_____

_____

_____

_____

_____

_____

_____

_____

_____

_____

_____

_____

_____

_____

_____

_____

_____

_____

_____

_____

Notes

_____

_____

_____

_____

_____

_____

_____

_____

_____

_____

_____

_____

_____

_____

_____

_____

_____

_____

_____

Notes

_____

_____

_____

_____

_____

_____

_____

_____

_____

_____

_____

_____

_____

_____

_____

_____

_____

_____

Notes

_____

_____

_____

_____

_____

_____

_____

_____

_____

_____

_____

_____

_____

_____

_____

_____

_____

_____

_____

Notes

_____

_____

_____

_____

_____

_____

_____

_____

_____

_____

_____

_____

_____

_____

_____

_____

_____

_____

Notes

_____

_____

_____

_____

_____

_____

_____

_____

_____

_____

_____

_____

_____

_____

_____

_____

_____

_____